Cardiac Emergencies

Cardiac Emergencies
A Pocket Guide

Jim Nolan MD MRCP
Consultant Cardiologist, Cardiothoracic Centre, North Staffordshire
Hospital, Stoke-on-Trent, UK

John Greenwood MBChB MRCP
BHF Research Fellow, Department of Cardiology,
St James' University Hospital, Leeds, UK

Alan Mackintosh MA MD FRCP
Consultant Cardiologist, Department of Cardiology,
St James' University Hospital, Leeds, UK

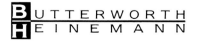

OXFORD BOSTON JOHANNESBURG MELBOURNE NEW DELHI SINGAPORE

Butterworth-Heinemann
Linacre House, Jordan Hill, Oxford OX2 8DP
225 Wildwood Avenue, Woburn, MA 01801-2041
A division of Reed Educational and Professional Publishing Ltd

 A member of the Reed Elsevier plc group

First published 1998

British Library Cataloguing in Publication Data
A catalogue record for this book is available from the British Library

Library of Congress Cataloguing in Publication Data
A catalogue record for this book is available from the Library of Congress

ISBN 0 7506 3833 8

Printed and bound in Great Britain by Biddles Ltd, Guildford & Kings Lynn
Typeset by David Gregson Associates, Beccles, Suffolk

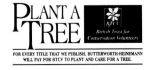

Contents

Preface

The first versions of this manuscript were written in the late 1980s and early 1990s. The principal stimulus for its subsequent development was provided by the consultants in the cardiology department at St James University Hospital in Leeds, who recognized the value of an up-to-date manuscript dealing with the management of common cardiac emergencies.

In this book we have aimed to produce concise evidence-based guidelines relating to the management of common cardiac emergencies for doctors and paramedical staff working in cardiology units, general medical units and related areas such as accident and emergency departments. Important references are provided at the end of each chapter for readers who wish to review the published evidence on which we have based our recommendations. We hope that the information is presented in a concise format that will allow easy access to the relevant information.

The text was developed with the input of many medical and paramedical staff. We would particularly like to thank Drs Philip Batin, Stephen Lindsey, Chris Pepper and Catherine Dickinson for their important and invaluable help. Finally we would like to thank Leslie Allsopp, Jane Lynch and Sue Macintosh for their help and support during the production of this manuscript.

Jim Nolan
John Greenwood
Alan Mackintosh

List of abbreviations

ACE:	angiotensin converting enzyme
AF:	atrial fibrillation
AICD:	automatic implantable cardioverter defibrillator
AII:	angiotensin II
APTT:	activated partial thromboplastin time
APSAC:	anistreplase
ARDS:	adult respiratory distress syndrome
AV:	atrioventricular
AVNRT:	atrioventricular nodal re-entry tachycardia
AVRT:	atrio-ventricular re-entry tachycardia
BP:	blood pressure
CABG:	coronary artery bypass grafting
CCU:	coronary care unit
COPD:	chronic obstructive pulmonary disease
CPAP:	continuous positive airways pressure
CPR:	cardiopulmonary resuscitation
CT:	computerized tomography
CXR:	chest x-ray
ECG:	electrocardiogram
EMD:	electromechanical dissociation
EP:	electrophysiology
EPS:	electrophysiological study
ESR:	erythrocyte sedimentation rate
ET:	endotracheal tube
FBC:	full blood count
GI:	gastrointestinal
GTN:	glyceryl trinitrate
HBDH:	hydroxy butyrate dehydrogenase
IABP:	intra-aortic balloon pump
IMH:	intramural haemorrhage
IV:	intravenous
JVP:	jugular venous pressure

LMWH:	low molecular weight heparin
LVF:	left ventricular failure
MI:	myocardial infarction
MRI:	magnetic resonance imaging
PA:	pulmonary artery
PAWP:	pulmonary artery wedge pressure
PE:	pulmonary embolism
PEEP:	positive end expiratory pressure
PTCA:	percutaneous transluminal coronary angioplasty
RA:	right atrium
RBBB:	right bundle branch block
RTA:	road traffic accident
rt-PA:	recombinant tissue, plasminogen activator
RV:	right ventricle
SLE:	systemic lupus erythematosis
SVC:	superior vena cava
TIA:	transient ischaemic attack
TOE:	transoesophageal echocardiogram
V/Q:	ventilation perfusion
VF:	ventricular fibrillation
VSD:	ventricular septal defect
VT:	ventricular tachycardia
WBC:	white blood cell count
WPW:	Wolff–Parkinson–White

1 The coronary care unit

Background

Coronary care units (CCUs) were developed in the 1960s when defibrillation became available. Subsequent developments such as temporary pacing and thrombolysis have reinforced the need for a specified unit. The aim of a CCU is to concentrate patients with life-threatening cardiac disorders in a properly organized area of the hospital staffed by appropriately trained doctors and nurses. The concentration of patients and resources allows ready access to equipment for diagnosing and treating these conditions and their complications.

Approximately one-third of patients with an acute cardiac ischaemic event will die in the community within one or two hours of the onset of their first symptoms, and a large proportion of these deaths are due to potentially reversible ventricular fibrillation. The outlook for these patients can only be improved by community resuscitation schemes, prevention, and education initiatives.

In the early 1960s, around 25 per cent of patients admitted to hospital with acute myocardial infarction (MI) died before discharge. The hospital mortality rate has now fallen to around 10 per cent in patients below 65 years of age, and this reduction in early mortality is due to therapeutic intervention with thrombolytic agents and aspirin. Beta-blockers, angiotensin converting enzyme (ACE) inhibitors, revascularization and better treatment of arrhythmias have all helped to improve the long-term prognosis of infarct survivors. Despite improvements in therapy, mortality from MI remains relatively high in the UK, with data from the recent GUSTO-III study suggesting that mortality in the UK is 30 per cent higher than in most other participating countries. This may reflect the relative underutilization of secondary prevention, rehabilitation and revascularization strategies in the UK.

The majority of deaths in patients with MI occur in the first 24 hours. Patients at particular risk of early death are the elderly, those with a previous or large MI, diabetics, and those who develop acute heart failure. Approximately 10 per cent of patients with acute MI who are admitted to a CCU will develop a life-threatening ventricular arrhythmia.

There is always a risk of sudden life-threatening ventricular arrhythmias in the first few post-infarct hours, even in a seemingly well patient, but these may be reversible if treated promptly and correctly. Many life-threatening ventricular arrhythmias occur in patients with well-preserved ventricular function, and the prognosis is good in these cases if appropriate treatment is received. When life-threatening ventricular arrhythmias occur in patients with impaired ventricular function and overt heart failure, the chances of successful resuscitation are much lower.

Following discharge from CCU, most patients do well, with 90 per cent surviving the first year. Those patients most likely to die in the first post-infarct year can now be identified by a series of clinical and investigational features, and medical intervention in these cases may improve the long-term prognosis (Chapter 15).

Guidelines for admission

Age is not a major factor in determining suitability for admission to CCU. If a patient requires rhythm monitoring, is likely to benefit from close supervision by appropriately trained medical and nursing staff, and is fit enough to be resuscitated should cardiac arrest supervene, then admission to CCU is appropriate. Particular patient groups who merit CCU admission are:

1. Patients with suspected or definite acute MI

2. Patients with suspected unstable angina

3. Patients with serious arrhythmias

4. Patients with severe heart failure.

If a patient requires admission but CCU is full, consider moving patients to free a bed. It is usually preferable to move a stable patient out of CCU rather than admit an unwell patient to a bed in a general ward.

Key points

- The CCU is an area where staff and equipment are concentrated to optimize the treatment of patients with acute cardiac conditions.

- One-third of patients with an acute MI die before reaching hospital.

- In-hospital mortality in younger patients has been substantially reduced since the early 1960s.

- Most in-hospital deaths occur in the first 24 hours, so this is the time when you need to be most vigilant.

- Most patients who survive their time on CCU do well, with 90 per cent surviving at least one year.

- Life-threatening ventricular arrhythmias occurring in the absence of severe impairment of ventricular function have a good prognosis with appropriate treatment. When they complicate severe ventricular impairment, prognosis is less favourable.

References

Brown, N., Young, T., Gray, D., *et al.* (1997). Inpatient deaths from acute myocardial infarction 1982–1992; analysis of data in the Nottingham heart attack register. *Br. Med. J.*, **315**, 159–164.

Evans, T. R. (1998). Cardiac arrests outside hospital. *Br. Med. J.*, **316**, 1031–2.

Hildebrandt, P., Jenson, G., Kober, C., *et al.* (1994). Myocardial infarction 1979–1988 in Denmark: Similar trends in age-related incidence, in-hospital mortality and complications. *Eur. Heart J.*, **15**, 877–881.

Jollis, J., Delong, E., Peterson, E., *et al.* (1996). Outcome of acute myocardial infarction according to the speciality of the admitting physician. *N. Eng. J. Med.*, **335**, 1880–1887.

Stevenson, R., Ranjadayalan, K., Wilkinson, P., *et al.* (1993). Short- and long-term prognosis of acute myocardial infarction since introduction of thrombolysis. *Br. Med. J.*, **307**, 349–353.

World Health Organization (1994). Myocardial infarction and coronary deaths in the World Organization MONICA project. Registration procedures, event rates and case fatality rates in 38 populations from 21 countries in 4 continents. *Circulation*, **90**, 583–612.

2

Pathophysiology of acute cardiac ischaemic syndromes

Background

Ischaemic heart disease is the most common cause of mortality in the United Kingdom, accounting for 30 per cent of all deaths. The most common syndromes seen in hospital practice are MI, unstable angina and heart failure.

Approximately 600 000 people in the United Kingdom are affected by an episode of major cardiac ischaemia (myocardial infarction or unstable angina) every year. Suspected or proven cardiac ischaemia is the commonest reason for medical admission to a general hospital. Following a peak in the mid-1960s, mortality from ischaemic heart disease has declined by around 30 per cent in the United Kingdom, and although the precise cause of this mortality reduction is unclear, it is likely that it is due to improvements in nutrition and lifestyle, and better risk factor management combined with improved diagnostic and management strategies.

Although there are many possible causes of cardiac ischaemia, it is most commonly due to luminal narrowing of the coronary arteries, associated with the development of coronary atheroma. Major risk factors predisposing to the development of coronary atheroma are:

1. Male sex
2. Increasing age
3. Family history
4. Smoking
5. Hyperlipidaemia
6. Hypertension
7. Diabetes mellitus.

Acute cardiac ischaemic syndromes represent a continuous spectrum of disease with the same underlying cause; the disruption of a stable atheromatous plaque to form an unstable lesion with superadded thrombus formation. Following disruption and fissuring of a plaque, platelet deposition, activation of the clotting cascade and release of vasoactive substances occur. The end result is narrowing of the coronary artery, and eventual occlusion (which may be intermittent). This leads to unstable angina or MI, depending on the duration of vessel occlusion, the size of the artery, the site of occlusion and the presence or absence of collateral vessels.

In recent years, much research has focused on the formation of the disrupted plaque and subsequent thrombus. Our knowledge has increased (for example, we know that a lipid-rich plaque is more vulnerable than a fibrous one), but we are a long way from understanding why a specific plaque ruptures at a specific moment. We now realize that there is only a loose correlation between the severity of the atheromatous narrowing and the risk of rupture. In general, severe narrowings are more vulnerable than mild ones, but the diseased coronary arteries contain many more mild narrowings than severe ones. It seems that the majority of acute ischaemic syndromes start with plaques which are producing no more than a 50 per cent stenosis, a degree of narrowing which would not normally produce symptoms or be regarded as a site for percutaneous transluminal coronary angioplasty (PTCA) or coronary artery bypass grafting (CABG).

Unstable angina

In unstable angina, plaque disruption is not usually as extensive as in patients with myocardial infarction, and total occlusion of the ischaemia-related artery is initially uncommon. Episodes of rest pain with associated ST segment changes develop, and may resolve as the morphology of the coronary artery alters. The process may progress and become irreversible, leading to total coronary occlusion and MI in a substantial proportion of patients over the following three months. Twelve month mortality is similar to that of patients admitted to hospital with acute MI.

Non-Q-wave infarction

Around 30 per cent of all patients admitted with acute MI do not develop Q-waves. In the early stages of non-Q-wave infarction, vessel occlusion may be total. Occlusions may occur distally, collateral blood flow is often good, and the time to spontaneous reperfusion is relatively short. Less myocardium is infarcted, and the necrosis is usually partial thickness only. It should be noted that although non-Q-wave infarcts are usually smaller than Q-wave infarcts, with a consequent lower early in-hospital mortality, the incidence of reinfarction is higher due to the persistence of an underlying unstable lesion which supplies viable myocardium. Overall mortality at one year is similar to that of Q-wave infarction.

An important sub-group of non-Q-wave infarcts is characterized by ST segment depression on the initial ECG. This group has a significant mortality rate in the first few weeks (higher than anterior Q-wave infarcts). The electrocardiographic appearances may reflect widespread coronary artery disease and/or pre-existing myocardial damage, both of which will increase the post-infarction mortality rate.

Q-wave infarction

In this condition, prolonged occlusion of a major coronary artery occurs. Collateral supply to the myocardium distal to the occlusion is usually poor, and a full-thickness area of myocardium infarcts. A large area of myocardium is usually involved, resulting in an extensive infarction. Such extensive full-thickness infarcts are associated with deleterious ventricular remodelling, leading to heart failure, ventricular arrhythmias and an adverse prognosis.

Therapeutic implications

Knowledge of the pathophysiology of acute cardiac ischaemic syndromes has helped to optimize drug treatment. Anticoagulants, aspirin and thrombolytic agents limit or reverse thrombus formation on unstable atheromatous plaques. Nitrates and beta-blockers reverse vasoconstriction and reduce myocardial oxygen consumption, limiting the harmful effects of vessel occlusion. Statins and ACE inhibitors stabilize atheromatous plaques, and thereby prevent the onset of acute ischaemic syndromes. Over the next decade, newer antiplatelet and anticoagulant agents such as hirudin and IIB/IIIA receptor antagonists may further improve our ability to prevent the progression of acute ischaemic syndromes. When an infarct does occur, ACE inhibitors help to prevent the detrimental ventricular remodelling which leads to heart failure.

Key points

- Ischaemic heart disease is the commonest cause of death in the UK.

- Plaque fissuring with consequent local activation of the clotting system and vasospasm is the cause of unstable angina and acute MI.

- Unstable angina, non-Q-wave infarction and Q-wave infarction represent a spectrum of disease with a similar 12 month mortality, once the acute phase is over.

References

Ambrose, J. A. (1992). Plaque disruption and the acute syndromes of unstable angina and myocardial infarction; if the substrate is similar, why is the clinical presentation different? *J. Am. Coll. Cardiol.*, **19**, 1653–1658.

Davies, M. J. and Thomas, A. C. (1985). Plaque fissuring – the cause of acute myocardial infarction, sudden ischaemic death, and crescendo angina. *Br. Heart J.*, **53**, 363–373.

Davies, M. J. and Woolf, N. (1993). Atherosclerosis: what is it and why does it occur? *Br. Heart J.*, **69**, 3–11.

Fuster, V., Badimon, L., Badimon, J. J., *et al.* (1992). The pathogenesis of coronary artery disease and the acute coronary syndromes. *N. Engl. J. Med.*, **326**, 242–250.

Sans, S., Kesteloot, H. and Kromhout, D. (1997). The burden of cardiovascular diseases mortality in Europe. *Eur. Heart J.*, **18**, 1231–1248.

Tunstall-Pedoe, H., Woodward, M., Tavendale, R., *et al.* (1997). Comparison of the prediction by 27 different factors of coronary heart disease and death in men and women of the Scottish Heart Health Study: cohort study. *Br. Med. J.*, **315**, 722–729.

Vortiainen, E., Puska, P., Pekkanen, J., *et al.* (1994). Changes in risk factors explain changes in mortality from ischaemic heart disease in Finland. *Br. Med. J.*, **309**, 23–27.

Zatonski, W. A., McMichael, A. J. and Powles, J. W. (1998). Ecological study of reasons for sharp decline in mortality from ischaemic heart disease in Poland since 1991. *Br. Med. J.*, **316**, 1047–1051.

3

Diagnosis in acute cardiac ischaemic syndromes

Background

Acute chest pain is a common reason for patients attending the accident and emergency department. Some of these patients have acute myocardial ischaemia, with a significant associated risk of death or serious complications. The outcome in these patients can be improved by appropriate therapy after admission to hospital. Many other patients have another non-cardiac cause for their chest pain, and often do not require admission. This chapter gives guidelines on diagnosing acute cardiac ischaemia and on differentiating it from other non-cardiac causes of chest pain.

As a general principle, patients with symptoms suggestive of myocardial ischaemia at rest lasting for more than 15 minutes should be admitted to hospital, even in the absence of changes in the electrocardiogram (ECG). Patients with evidence of acute MI or unstable angina should preferably be admitted to CCU, but if transfer is likely to be delayed, appropriate treatment should be commenced in the emergency department.

Acute myocardial infarction

The diagnosis of acute MI is usually made in a patient with cardiac ischaemic pain that occurs at rest, lasts for more than 15 minutes, and is accompanied by diagnostic electrocardiographic and enzyme changes.

Clinical features

The pain of cardiac ischaemia is typically retrosternal, severe, crushing, radiates to the neck, arms or back, and is associated with nausea, vomiting and sweating, related to the release of toxins from injured myocardial cells and autonomic activation.

Remember that:

1. The pain can be atypical (epigastric, sited in the neck, arms or back only, or unusual in character) and, particularly with inferior infarcts, can be difficult to distinguish from dyspepsia.

2. The pain can be minimal or absent, especially in the elderly or diabetic.

3. For each individual, cardiac pain may vary in intensity and radiation, but it is broadly similar in character and position on each occasion. Ask the patient to compare the pain with any earlier, proven, ischaemic attacks, including classical angina. If the patient feels that the pain is similar, then even atypical symptoms are probably cardiac in origin.

Physical examination is unremarkable in most patients with acute myocardial infarction, apart from the presence of anxiety, sweating and a tachycardia. Signs of heart failure or hypotension occur in patients with extensive ventricular damage. Rhythm abnormalities may be obvious in some patients.

Electrocardiographic changes

The ECG is seldom completely normal in a patient with acute MI. The typical changes of acute MI are:

1. *ST elevation in the leads overlying the area of infarction.* This can develop within minutes of the onset of infarction, and may persist. Persistence after the first few hours is often associated with failure to reperfuse the occluded coronary artery and the development of ventricular dilatation.

2. *Pathological Q-waves in the leads overlying the area of infarction.* Q-waves are usually associated with full thickness MI, develop within a few hours of the onset of the infarct and usually persist long-term. In a few patients, Q-waves can regress. Associated with the development of Q-waves is a reduction of the R-wave amplitude in affected leads.

3. *T-wave inversion in the leads overlying the area of infarction.* This develops as the ST elevation subsides, and usually resolves over 7–14 days. The first sign of infarction may be the development of tall, peaked T-waves in the area overlying the infarct zone.

The distribution of ECG changes provides some information on the area of myocardium involved, for example:

- Changes in V2–V6 indicate extensive anterolateral MI due to proximal occlusion of a large left anterior descending artery (Figure 3.1). These patients usually suffer extensive full thickness infarction, and are at

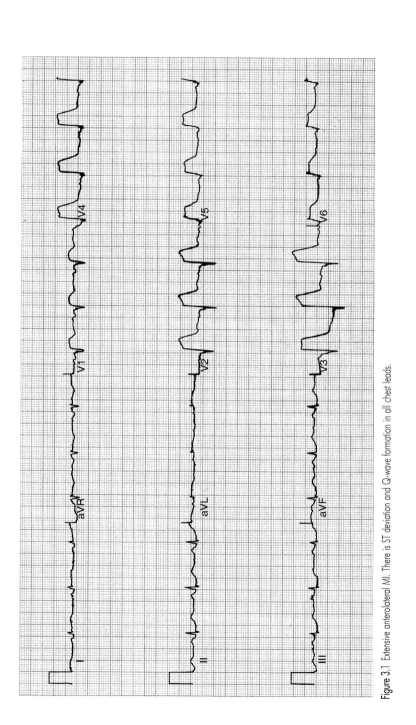

Figure 3.1 Extensive anterolateral MI. There is ST deviation and Q-wave formation in all chest leads.

increased risk of arrhythmias, heart failure, mechanical complications and early death.

- Changes in V2–V4 indicate septal infarction, usually associated with more distal occlusion of a well-collateralized left anterior descending artery or one of its branches. These patients usually sustain a smaller infarct, with a lower risk of complications and a better prognosis.

- Changes in I, aVL, V5 and V6 indicate lateral infarction, due to occlusion of the circumflex artery or the diagonal branch of the left anterior descending (Figure 3.2). These patients usually sustain a relatively limited infarct with a lower risk of complications and a better prognosis.

- Changes in II, III, and aVF indicate inferior infarction, usually due to occlusion of the right coronary artery (Figure 3.3). Patients with inferior infarction have a relatively low incidence of heart failure and tachyarrhythmias, but an increased incidence of bradyarrhythmias (because the AV node is principally supplied by the right coronary artery in 90 per cent of patients). Patients with inferior infarction generally have a good prognosis, although those with very extensive infarction (indicated by the presence of changes in the inferior, lateral and posterior leads) are a high risk subgroup. Hypotension in patients with inferior infarction may be due to right ventricular involvement; these patients respond well to intravenous (IV) fluids and have a good prognosis, unlike patients with hypotension due to extensive left ventricular impairment (see Chapter 11).

- Tall R-waves in V1–V3 may be due to an accessory pathway, right bundle branch block (RBBB) or right ventricular hypertrophy. Tall R-waves in V1–V3 associated with ST depression in these leads in a patient with a history of ischaemic chest pain suggest posterior MI (Figure 3.4). This can often be difficult to diagnose, but serial changes developing in ECGs repeated at regular intervals are highly suggestive, and indicate the need to proceed with thrombolytic therapy.

A large infarct is indicated by the presence of changes in several leads, and marked ST segment elevation.

Some patients present with a story highly suggestive of intermittent episodes of cardiac ischaemia at rest, but a normal or equivocal ECG. These patients should be admitted for observation, especially if the symptoms are new, since they may have either unstable angina or an evolving infarct. However, they do represent a low-risk group.

A rise in creatine kinase over the first 48 hours after an episode of chest pain provides biochemical evidence of an acute infarct. HBDH levels remain elevated for several days after infarction, and are therefore useful in making a retrospective diagnosis if necessary.

To diagnose infarction, the rise in the creatine kinase should be to at least

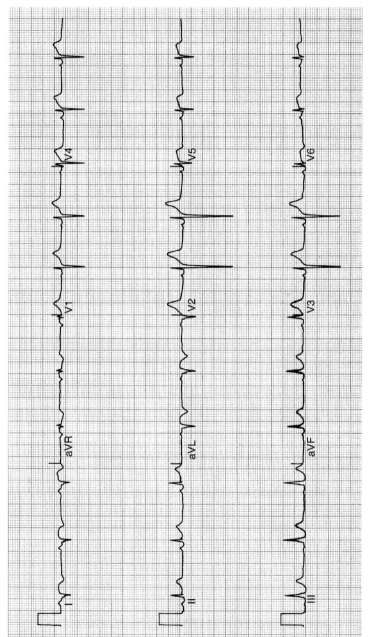

Figure 3.2 Lateral MI. There is evolving ST elevation, T-wave inversion and Q-wave formation in leads I, aVL, V5 and V6.

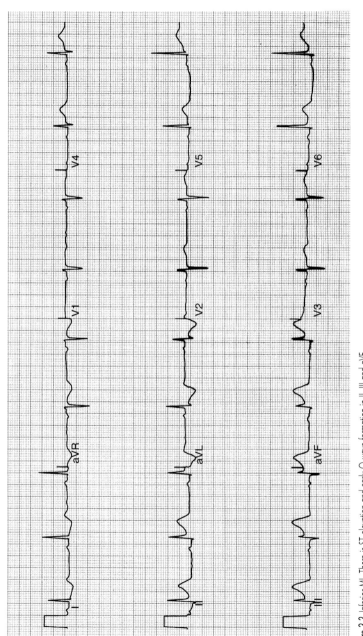

Figure 3.3 Inferior MI. There is ST elevation and early Q-wave formation in II, III and aVF.

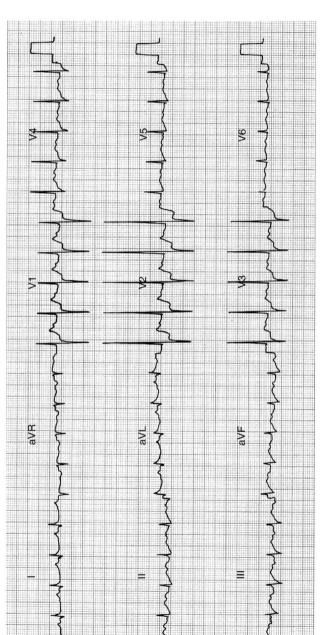

Figure 3.4 Posterior MI. Tall R-waves with associated ST depression in V1–V3.

twice the upper limit of normal. However, creatine kinase can be released by any muscle in the body and is not specific to heart muscle, therefore many non-cardiac illnesses can produce a modest rise in the enzyme. Extreme caution is needed in diagnosing an MI from an enzyme rise without suggestive acute ECG changes.

The creatine kinase MB fraction is more specific for cardiac muscle damage, but it is not universally available and does not always supply the expected clear result. A borderline total kinase level may be accompanied by a borderline MB fraction.

Unstable angina

Patients with unstable angina develop episodes of cardiac ischaemic pain. This is similar in site and nature to the pain of stable angina or myocardial infarction, and symptoms may:

1. Occur at rest or on minimal exertion

2. Be unresponsive to the patient's normal treatment (e.g. unresponsive to GTN in normal doses)

3. Occur with increasing frequency

4. Be prolonged (whereas usually episodes last less than 30 minutes).

Typically, the ECG recorded during an episode of pain shows ST depression in the territory of the involved coronary artery. Serial ECGs show no ST elevation or Q-wave development, and cardiac enzymes are not elevated unless the unstable angina progresses to a full-blown infarction. The ECG diagnosis of unstable angina depends on finding transient ST segment or T-wave changes associated with the presenting symptoms.

Variant angina due to dominant coronary spasm is very rare, and is associated with episodic ST elevation, T-wave peaking and pseudo-normalization of T-waves during episodes of pain. Coronary spasm can occur at any time, and symptoms therefore often do not bear any relationship to exertion.

Other causes of chest pain

Non-cardiac chest pain can arise from:

1. The aorta in acute dissection. The pain of aortic dissection is severe and of sudden onset; it is tearing in nature, often radiates to the back, and

may be associated with hypertension, aortic regurgitation, neurological signs and pulse deficits (see Chapter 20).

2. The pleura in pneumonia, pulmonary embolism or pneumothorax. Pain arising from the pleura is unilateral, sharp and stabbing, and worse on inspiration. There may be associated signs of pneumonia, pulmonary embolus or deep venous thrombosis. The majority of patients with pulmonary embolus have no ECG changes apart from a tachycardia or atrial fibrillation. ECG changes of $S_1Q_3T_3$ or right heart strain are associated with large emboli and are often transient and easily missed. In spontaneous pneumothorax, there may be central chest pain with few auscultatory signs. Spontaneous pneumothorax is a strong possibility in patients with chronic obstructive pulmonary disease (COPD), who present with chest pain and dyspnoea in the absence of ECG evidence of acute myocardial ischaemia. A chest x-ray (CXR) is vital to rule out the presence of air in the pleural space.

3. The upper GI tract in oesophageal reflux or peptic ulcer disease. Dyspeptic pain arising from the upper GI tract is usually burning in nature, may have a clear relationship to posture or food, and is often relieved by antacids. Oesophageal pain may, however, be very similar to the pain of cardiac ischaemia. Exercise-induced oesophageal pain mimicking angina has been well described. In some individuals, oesophageal spasm may occur in association with ST segment change. Nitrates and calcium antagonists will relieve the pain of oesophageal spasm. Correct diagnosis in these difficult patients requires coronary anteriography, investigations to rule out coronary spasm, myocardial perfusion imaging and ambulatory oesophageal pH and pressure monitoring. Pain due to ischaemia of the inferior surface of the heart often mimics dyspepsia.

4. The pericardium in pericarditis. Pericardial pain is retrosternal, sharp, eased by sitting forward, and may worsen with inspiration. It is commonly seen post-infarction, or in a young adult with acute post-viral pericarditis. A pericardial rub is common, although it may be intermittent. Diagnostic concave ST elevation may be present in patients with post-viral pericarditis.

5. The bones and muscles in musculoskeletal disorders. Musculoskeletal chest pain is usually unilateral, localized and sharp. It is exacerbated by movement or local pressure. There may be a history of trauma.

6. The skin in acute dermatological conditions. Acute skin conditions can (rarely) produce chest pain. The unilateral pain of shingles precedes the rash, and may confuse the unwary.

7. Outside the chest cavity, for example, referred pain from the gall bladder or neck. Pain due to gall bladder disease may show a clear relationship to food, and be associated with abdominal signs. Pain

referred from the cervical or thoracic spine will have features of musculoskeletal chest pain.

Key points

- Acute MI is easily diagnosed when typical pain coexists with clear-cut ECG changes. *A normal resting ECG does not exclude the presence of significant coronary artery disease.*

- Pain and ECG changes may be atypical. If you are in doubt about the diagnosis, admit the patient for further evaluation.

- There are many non-cardiac causes of chest pain. Careful history taking will allow differentiation in many cases.

- Patients with extensive anterolateral infarction are at high risk of heart failure, tachyarrhythmias and mechanical complications.

- Patients with inferior infarction are at high risk of bradyarrhythmic complications.

References

Adam, J., Trent, R. and Rawles, J. on behalf of the GREAT Group (1993). Earliest electrocardiographic evidence of myocardial infarction: implications for thrombolytic therapy. *Br. Med. J.*, **307**, 409–413.

Grijseels, E. W. M., Decloers, J. W., Hoes, A. W., *et al.* (1995) Pre-hospital triage of patients with suspected acute myocardial infarction. *Eur. Heart J.*, **16**, 325–332.

Hlatky, M. A. (1997). Evaluation of chest pain in the emergency department. *N. Engl. J. Med.*, **337**, 1687–1689.

4

Emergency and early care of acute myocardial infarction

Background

Patients with evolving MI often do not request medical aid until symptoms have been present for more than one hour. This patient delay occurs at the most critical time in the course of the illness, when pain is often severe and the risk of ventricular tachyarrhythmias and cardiac arrest is high. Although mass public education campaigns may shorten the duration of this patient delay, they have had no significant impact on outcome. Once a patient with suspected acute MI arrives in hospital, rapid processing is necessary to establish an early diagnosis and allow effective emergency care to be instituted.

Patients who present to the emergency department with possible acute MI should be reviewed as soon as possible by an appropriately trained doctor. The initial assessment should be rapid, and aimed at establishing the diagnosis, assessing the haemodynamic state and determining suitability for reperfusion therapy. Comprehensive history taking and examination can be deferred until the patient has received appropriate emergency care and is stable on CCU. Patients with clear-cut clinical features of acute MI and an ECG that demonstrates ST elevation or bundle branch block should enter a 'fast track' system, designed to ensure that they receive appropriate emergency care and that thrombolytic therapy is instituted within 90 minutes of the initial call for medical assistance. A successful fast track system is only possible if medical staff respond rapidly to calls from the emergency department, and you should aim to review patients with a suggestive history and ECG changes within ten minutes of their arrival in the emergency department. The 'door-to-needle' time should not exceed 20 minutes for fast track patients.

Emergency care

In a patient with chest pain lasting for more than 15 minutes and not responding to sublingual nitrates, and with electrocardiographic ST elevation or left bundle branch block, a provisional diagnosis of acute myocardial infarction can confidently be reached. If the clinical features are atypical and the ECG is equivocal but there is a strong suspicion of evolving myocardial infarction, treatment with heparin, beta-blockers, nitrates and aspirin should be instituted. The patient should be admitted to CCU, and repeated ECG recordings or, if available, continuous ST segment monitoring performed. If ST segment elevation or bundle branch block develops, thrombolytic therapy should be administered. Thrombolytic therapy should not be given to patients with a normal ECG, T-wave inversion or ST depression; there is no evidence that lytic therapy will be of benefit in these cases.

Having reached a provisional diagnosis of acute MI, emergency care consists of relief of pain, breathlessness and anxiety, and administration of thrombolytic therapy and aspirin as early as possible. The priorities are to:

1. Establish venous access with a large-bore cannula in an arm vein, providing ready access for drug administration, and to institute rhythm monitoring to aid in the rapid detection and treatment of arrhythmias.

2. Provide adequate analgesia, which is vital. Uncontrolled pain and anxiety is associated with sympathetic activation, with resultant detrimental effects on cardiac performance, oxygen consumption and the arrhythmia threshold. Intravenous opioids are indicated to provide rapid relief of pain. Intramuscular injections should be avoided, as they have a slower onset of action, are associated with unpredictable absorption, may cause a haematoma if thrombolytic therapy is given, and can affect CK estimations. The agent of choice is diamorphine 2.5–5.0 mg by slow IV injection, with metroclopramide 10 mg IV as an anti-emetic. The dose should be repeated every five minutes until adequate analgesia is achieved. If repeated administration of diamorphine fails to relieve the pain, consider intravenous beta-blockers or nitrates. Respiratory depression produced by diamorphine can, if necessary, be rapidly reversed by naloxone.

3. Treat pulmonary oedema with IV frusemide 40–80 mg.

4. Provide supplemental oxygen. Hypoxia is common in patients with evolving infarction, and may increase myocardial necrosis or have adverse metabolic effects. Supplemental oxygen will optimize oxygen delivery and limit ischaemia, and should be given to all patients with breathlessness or features of heart failure. Since hypoxia may be present

in 20 per cent of patients with an initially uncomplicated infarct, pulse oximetry should be instituted in all cases, and oxygen given if saturation falls below 93 per cent. High concentration (up to 60 per cent) oxygen can be given via an MC mask if necessary. If the patient has COPD, commence therapy with 24 or 28 per cent oxygen via a ventimask, and adjust the concentration depending on blood gas measurements to prevent CO_2 retention in patients who are reliant on hypoxic drive to maintain ventilation.

5. Commence treatment with thrombolytic therapy and aspirin (in an initial dose of at least 160 mg) in the emergency department. It is important to commence thrombolytic therapy as early as possible. Mortality in patients treated within an hour of the onset of symptoms is only 1.2 per cent, compared to 8.7 per cent for those treated later.

Having established intravenous access and continuous rhythm monitoring and administered analgesia, oxygen, aspirin and thrombolytic therapy, the patient can be transferred to the CCU for further evaluation and therapy.

Early investigation and treatment on the CCU

Following transfer to CCU a full history and examination can be performed. The indications for intravenous beta-blockers (Chapter 6) and urgent PTCA (Chapter 7) should be reviewed. Obtain urgent electrolytes, glucose, blood count and CXR. Send blood for routine estimation of cardiac enzymes and cholesterol. A variety of additional treatment options have recently been evaluated, and this section discusses their relative merits and the indications for use.

Hypokalaemia

Hypokalaemia is common in patients with acute infarction, and is related to prior treatment with diuretics or catecholamine effects on electrolyte handling. Hypokalaemia is associated with myocardial electrical instability (the incidence of VF may be as high as 15 per cent in infarcts associated with a potassium of 3.0–3.5 mmol/l, and 5 per cent or less in infarcts associated with a potassium of 4.5–5.0 mmol/l) and should be corrected. If the serum potassium is below 4.0 mmol/l, supplements should be given. In the presence of an arrhythmia, administer intravenous potassium as detailed in Chapter 24.

The serum potassium should be re-checked after an interval of two to three hours to ensure that a level above 4.0 mmol/l has been achieved. If serum potassium is below 4.0 mmol/l in the absence of an important arrhythmia, then give oral potassium supplements (e.g. SLOW K, three tablets three times daily, providing approximately 120 mmol of potassium daily) and recheck potassium after 12 to 18 hours.

Magnesium therapy

A number of small and early studies (including LIMIT-2) suggested that routine administration of magnesium may reduce mortality following acute infarction by the beneficial effects on heart rate, contractility, electrical stability and platelet activity. The routine use of magnesium was therefore examined in almost 60 000 patients in ISIS-4, and this showed that treatment had no beneficial effect on mortality. Subgroup analysis showed no benefit, even when magnesium was given early, or to patients who did not receive thrombolytic therapy. There is therefore no evidence to support the routinue use of magnesium in patients with evolving acute myocardial infarction. Magnesium is, however, still indicated for the treatment of arrhythmias as detailed in Chapters 8 and 18.

Nitrate therapy

Nitrates have a number of potentially beneficial effects (systemic vaso-dilatation and coronary artery dilatation), and meta-analysis of small early studies suggested that their routine administration to patients with acute infarction may reduce mortality. The ISIS-4 and GISSI-3 trials investigated routine nitrate use in a total of almost 80 000 patients, and found no beneficial effect on mortality. Although nitrates are safe and effective in the treatment of post-infarction ischaemia or heart failure, they should not routinely be administered to uncomplicated patients.

Hyperglycaemia

Patients with pre-existing diabetes have an increased risk of ischaemic heart disease, and an unfavourable prognosis following acute myocardial infarction. Patients who have no history of diabetes but an elevated glucose on admission also have a poor prognosis. The high mortality may be related to the occurrence of autonomic neuropathy, pre-existing ventricular dysfunction or due to detrimental myocardial cellular changes induced by diabetes. Additionally, sympathetic activation will induce insulin resistance and hyperglycaemia in susceptible patients, increasing the release of non-esterified fatty acids, which augment myocardial oxygen consumption, depress contractility and increase the risk of heart failure. A strategy of controlling elevated plasma glucose by insulin infusion followed by subcutaneous injections in hyperglycaemic patients with acute myocardial infarction could prevent these adverse metabolic effects, and was investigated in over 600 patients randomized in the DIGAMI trial. Treatment with intravenous insulin in patients with an admission glucose >11 mmol/l reduced early and late (three year) mortality by around 30 per cent. The maximum reduction in mortality occurred in patients who had not previously received insulin therapy, and were at low risk of death on the basis of clinical criteria. On the basis of this trial data, it is recommended that all patients with an admission glucose >11 mmol/l should be commenced on a sliding scale intravenous insulin infusion (Chapter 24) with the infusion rate adjusted to maintain blood glucose in the range 7–11 mmol/l, in combination with 500 ml of 5% dextrose infused over 24 hours. Oral hypoglycaemic agents should be withdrawn. The infusion should be continued for at least 24 hours, or until the patient is clinically stable, and followed by at least three months' treatment with subcutaneous insulin.

Prophylactic antiarrhythmic therapy

Prophylactic lignocaine can reduce the incidence of ventricular arrhythmias in the acute phase of acute MI. Unfortunately, it also increases the risk of asystole, and this offsets its beneficial effect on ventricular arrhythmias. Since it has no overall beneficial effect on mortality, the routine use of prophylactic antiarrhythmic therapy with lignocaine is not indicated.

Pre-existing drug therapy

Patients admitted with evolving acute MI are often already on treatment with oral beta-blockers for pre-existing angina or hypertension. Given the beneficial effects of beta-blockers following infarction and the potential adverse effects associated with abrupt beta-blocker withdrawal, administration of these agents should continue uninterrupted unless important heart failure or a symptomatic bradyarrhythmia develop.

Combined oral contraceptives are associated with an increased risk of thromboembolism and should be withdrawn.

Hormone replacement therapy reduces the risk of cardiac events in post-menopausal females, and should be continued without interruption in patients with evolving acute MI.

Key points

- It is important to review patients with suspected evolving acute MI as soon as possible after they arrive in the emergency department.

- Initial assessment should be rapid, and aimed at establishing the diagnosis and instituting appropriate emergency treatment.

- The priorities for emergency care in patients with evolving acute MI are the relief of pain and anxiety, the treatment of breathlessness, and the prompt administration of aspirin and thrombolytic therapy.

- Following admission to the CCU, it is important to obtain urgent electrolytes and glucose, and institute appropriate corrective therapy.

References

Madias, J. E. and Hood, W. B. (1976). Reduction of precordial ST segment elevation in patients with anterior myocardial infarction by oxygen breathing. *Circulation*, **53**, 198–201.

Nattrass, M. (1997). Managing diabetics after myocardial infarction. Time for a more aggressive approach. *Br. Med. J.*, **314**, 1497.

Nordrehaug, J. E. and Lippe, G. V. D. (1983). Hypokalaemia and ventricular fibrillation in acute myocardial infarction. *Br. Heart. J.*, **50**, 525–529.

Rude, R. E., Poole, W. K., Muller, J. E., *et al.* (1983). Electrocardiographic and clinical criteria for recognition of acute myocardial infarction based on analysis of 3697 patients. *Am. J. Cardiol.*, **52**, 936–942.

Sullivan, J. M. (1996). Practical aspects of preventing and managing atherosclerotic disease in post-menopausal women. *Eur. Heart. J.*, **17** (Suppl. D), 32–37.

The Task Force on the Management of Acute Myocardial Infarction of the European Society of Cardiology. (1996). Acute myocardial infarction: pre-hospital and in-hospital management. *Eur. Heart. J.*, **17**, 43–63.

Weston, C. F. M., Penny, W. J. and Julian, D. G. (1994). Guidelines for the early management of patients with myocardial infarction. *Br. Med. J.*, **308**, 767–771.

Yusuf, S. and Flather, M. (1995). Magnesium in acute myocardial infarction. *Br. Med. J.*, **310**, 751–752.

5　Thrombolysis

Background

Large scale clinical trials have clearly demonstrated that the early administration of thrombolysis saves lives in acute MI. However, the magnitude of benefit is time dependent. Treatment within an hour of onset of symptoms is associated with a 50 per cent reduction in mortality; up to 12 hours after the onset of chest pain there is still a significant (though much smaller) reduction in mortality; and at 12–24 hours, a summary of the trials of 'delayed' thrombolysis has shown a trend towards reduction in mortality, but this failed to reach significance. Further studies in this area are warranted, as there may be patient subgroups who could benefit from late treatment. Thrombolysis is beneficial regardless of age, sex or infarct site. In addition, the administration of aspirin has an additive effect. Approximately 60 per cent of patients with acute MI are eligible for thrombolysis; 15 per cent have a contraindication, 15 per cent present late and 10 per cent have an initially non-diagnostic ECG.

On the basis of this data, thrombolysis should be considered for all patients presenting within 12 hours after the onset of chest pain and who have ST segment elevation or new bundle branch block on their ECG. There is no evidence of benefit from the administration of thrombolysis to patients with normal ECGs or ST segment depression at presentation. In these circumstances, the ECG should be repeated at regular intervals, or continuous ST segment monitoring instituted. If the criteria for thrombolysis are not fulfilled in a patient presenting with prolonged cardiac chest pain and ST segment depression, management should be along the lines outlined in Chapter 17 for unstable angina. Limiting thrombolysis in this fashion will reduce the risk of side-effects in patients with little potential for benefit.

Although new thrombolytic agents are under development, only the following treatments are currently licensed for acute MI in the UK: streptokinase, recombinant tissue plasminogen activator (rt-PA), anistreplase (APSAC) and reteplase. The former three agents were compared in the ISIS-3 study, which showed no overall difference in therapeutic efficacy using standard administration protocols. Therefore, on the basis of cost and similar efficacy, streptokinase is the first line treatment in the majority of cases. In certain circumstances (hypotension on admission, previous administration of streptokinase), rt-PA is preferable as it is less likely to cause a further fall in blood pressure and is effective even when streptokinase-neutralizing antibodies are present. Additionally, some patients will have a better prognosis if treated with rt-PA. The first GUSTO study examined an 'accelerated' regime of rt-PA administration, and showed an advantage in terms of mortality and early coronary artery patency, at the cost of a small increase in haemorrhagic stroke. With subgroup analysis of the first GUSTO trial, it is evident that the greatest benefit of rt-PA over streptokinase was in three subgroups (patients with anterior MIs, those aged less than 75 years, and those who presented within four hours of the onset of chest pain), and targeting these particular patients will optimize the cost effectiveness of rt-PA therapy.

Current investigative strategies are aimed at optimizing thrombolytic therapy for acute MI, in order to achieve early and complete reperfusion of the infarct-related artery. Establishment of normal blood flow in this vessel (TIMI grade 3) has been shown to be the most important correlate with clinical outcome. Mortality in patients who fail to achieve adequate flow in the infarct-related artery is ten times higher than in those who successfully re-establish adequate antegrade flow in the infarct-related artery. In addition to salvage of acutely ischaemic myocardium, a patent infarct-related artery helps to prevent ventricular remodeling leading to later heart failure and arrhythmias. The newest thrombolytic agent to be licensed for acute MI, reteplase, has been shown in small numbers of patients to have efficacy at least equivalent to that of streptokinase. Its potential advantage over other thrombolytic regimes may lie in its potential to restore TIMI grade 3 flow in more patients, and its simple administration as a non-weight adjusted, double IV bolus. This hypothesis was tested in the GUSTO-III trial. Over 15 000 patients with acute MI were randomized to either reteplase or accelerated rt-PA. Reteplase did not provide any additional survival benefit over accelerated rt-PA in the treatment of acute MI in GUSTO-III.

Although the search for superior thrombolytics will continue, significant advances in vessel patency may be achieved with improved adjuvant therapy. Although direct-acting antithrombins have been disappointing, platelet IIb/IIIa inhibitors have great promise. Despite these advances, it remains of fundamental importance to reduce the time delay between the onset of symptoms and the initiation of therapy. Every effort should be made to streamline pre-hospital and in-hospital procedures, which should be the subject of regular audit. The target 'door-to-needle' time of 20 minutes or less should not be an unobtainable goal.

Inclusion criteria

Patients suitable for thrombolysis are selected on the basis of the following criteria. The chosen thrombolytic agent should be administered without delay, and aspirin should be given in all cases.

1. Presentation within 12 hours of the onset of ischaemic cardiac pain in a patient with:
   a. ST segment elevation of at least 2 mm in two adjacent chest leads
   b. ST segment elevation of 1 mm in two adjacent limb leads
   c. true posterior infarction or new bundle branch block

2. Presentation 12–24 hours after onset of pain in the presence of ongoing symptoms and ECG evidence of evolving infarction.

Exclusion criteria

These continue to evolve, and are in general decreasing as our experience with thrombolytic agents increases. At present there are few *absolute* contraindications. Many are now regarded as *relative*, to be interpreted within the clinical context. Criteria include:

1. Known coagulation disorder, including uncontrolled anticoagulation therapy
2. Active peptic ulceration, varices or recent GI haemorrhage (dyspepsia alone is not a contraindication)
3. Severe hypertension; systolic >200 mmHg and/or diastolic >110 mmHg
4. Traumatic cardiopulmonary resuscitation (CPR) (CPR performed by trained staff is no longer regarded as a contraindication)
5. Recent internal bleeding from any site (menstruation is not an absolute contraindication)
6. History of stroke with residual neurological deficit at any time, or TIA within three months
7. Surgery, major trauma or head injury within the last month

8. Pregnancy
9. Diabetic retinopathy (now only a relative contraindication, as the risk of intraocular bleeding is very small and the potential benefit of thrombolysis in diabetics far outweighs this risk).

If in doubt about administering thrombolysis, a senior colleague should be consulted. If risks outweigh the perceived benefits, primary PTCA is a safe and effective alternative.

Administration regime and indications for streptokinase

In the absence of contraindications, and if the patient does not fulfil the criteria for rt-PA, this is the drug of choice. Heparin with streptokinase has not been shown to have any clear beneficial effect, and will increase the risk of bleeding complications. Heparin is therefore not routinely given after streptokinase.

Administration of streptokinase: 1.5 MU in 100 ml normal saline over one hour.

Administration regime and indications for rt-PA

The indications for administering rt-PA in preference to streptokinase are:
1. Anterior infarction in patient < 75 years, presenting within four hours after onset of pain
2. Persistent hypotension < 90 mmHg systolic (streptokinase may exacerbate hypotension)
3. Administration of streptokinase more than four days previously (due to the formation of neutralizing antibodies, which may persist in 50 per cent of patients even after four years)
4. Previous documented severe allergic reaction in response to streptokinase.

Accelerated rt-PA is given as a 15 mg IV bolus, followed by 0.75 mg/kg (to a maximum of 50 mg) over 30 minutes, followed by 0.5 mg/kg (up to 35 mg) over one hour (see Table 5.1).

As rt-PA has a short half-life there is increased potential for early re-occlusion, and in general heparin is given intravenously for at least 24 hours, as:
1. 5000 unit bolus prior to the bolus of rt-PA
2. Following rt-PA administration, a continuous infusion of 1000 units per hour (adjusted according to APTT after six hours).

Table 5.1 Administration regime for rt-PA

Weight (kg)	50	60	70+
IV Bolus	15 mg	15 mg	15 mg
Infusion (30 minutes)	35 mg	45 mg	50 mg
Infusion (60 minutes)	25 mg	30 mg	35 mg

Complications

1. *Allergy.* Allergic reactions to streptokinase are due to the effect of pre-existing antistreptococcal antibodies. Mild urticarial reactions are the most common allergic response, and should be treated with 200 mg of IV hydrocortisone and 10 mg of IV chlorpheniramine. If a more severe reaction with bronchospasm occurs, 250–500 mcg of intramuscular adrenaline should be administered along with nebulized bronchodilators. Major anaphylaxis is very rare (0.1 per cent). If this occurs, with associated cardiovascular collapse, 5 ml of 1:10 000 adrenaline IV is first line therapy, followed by rapid volume loading with IV plasma expanders, steroids and antihistamines.

2. *Haemorrhage.* Minor bleeding at venepuncture sites is relatively common (3–4 per cent), but rarely requires any specific therapy other than direct compression at the site. Major haemorrhagic episodes requiring transfusion are rare (0.3 per cent). If a major bleed occurs:
   a. Stop thrombolytic infusion (or heparin)
   b. Reverse heparin with protamine sulphate
   c. Give two units of fresh frozen plasma immediately
   d. Give tranexamic acid 10 mg/kg by slow IV injection.

3. *Hypotension.* Hypotensive reactions to thrombolytic infusion can occur with any agent, but are more common with streptokinase. They should be treated initially by tilting the patient head down and, in the case of streptokinase, the infusion should be slowed down or if necessary halted for five minutes. It can usually be successfully restarted when the blood pressure (BP) recovers. Atropine 0.6 mg IV can be given if a bradycardia is also present. If the hypotension persists and is clearly associated with the infusion, then the drug should be stopped, and rt-PA substituted for streptokinase, as it is less likely to cause hypotension. In the case of severe persistent hypotension, fluids and inotropes can be administered cautiously if necessary.

4. *Cerebrovascular events.* The overall incidence of stroke is increased by only 0.1 per cent, since thrombolytic therapy causes a slight increase in cerebral haemorrhages which is offset by a reduction in cerebral infarcts. Use of rt-PA is associated with a greater risk of haemorrhagic stroke than

streptokinase. Stroke is more common in older patients. Treatment should be along the lines of those for major haemorrhage (as above). A CT head scan and neurological opinion may be helpful in determining treatment and prognosis.

Management after thrombolysis

Management of patients after thrombolysis should be along conventional lines, as outlined in Chapters 6–15. In particular, consideration should be given to the administration of IV beta-blockers for selected individuals, as they reduce the incidence of myocardial rupture. This section will focus on specific problems in the infarct-related artery. As discussed earlier, patency in this vessel is a powerful predictor of mortality, and at present thrombolytics achieve adequate patency in less than 60 per cent of patients. This is partly as a consequence of failure to reperfuse, and partly due to re-occlusion.

Failure to reperfuse

There are few accurate markers of successful reperfusion. Probably the best are the prompt resolution of chest pain, and reduction in ST segment elevation. Patients with persistent ST elevation 3 hours after the initiation of thrombolysis have a 17.5% mortality, compared with 2.5% in those with early resolution of ST elevation. Both of these are somewhat insensitive and non-specific, and a more quantitative correlate of reperfusion may be gained from cardiac enzyme release (e.g. creatinine kinase, CK-MB mass, myoglobin, troponin-T). However, frequent estimation of levels may be required, and at present early serial enzyme measurements are impractical for routine use in many units. Arrhythmias (commonly idioventricular rhythm) may be a sign of successful reperfusion, but are common after acute infarction and so cannot be regarded as a specific sign.

Patients with clinical evidence of failure to reperfuse (e.g. continuing pain, persisting/worsening ST segment elevation) 90 minutes after administration of thrombolysis, especially in the presence of haemodynamic instability, have a poor prognosis. Optimal management strategies are unclear at the present time, but include:

1. Invasive revascularization (e.g. rescue PTCA)
2. Further doses of thrombolytic therapy. For rescue thrombolysis, IV accelerated rt-PA is preferable to streptokinase, since it has a superior rate of re-establishing flow in the infarct-related artery

The options chosen will depend on clinical factors, local expertise and experience, and patients should be discussed with a senior colleague. For haemodynamically stable patients with a small infarct (ST elevation in <3 leads) the risks of rescue PTCA or thrombolysis probably outweigh the benefits, and a conservative approach is justified. For patients with large infarcts (marked ST elevation in multiple leads or haemodynamic instability) in whom failure to reperfuse is documented early (within the first 3–4 hours) then a rescue procedure stands a reasonable chance of re-establishing adequate perfusion, salvaging myocardium and improving prognosis. When failure to reperfuse is detected later, even re-establishment of flow in the occluded artery may not be beneficial, since there may be occlusion of the capillary circulation in the territory of the infarct-related artery.

Re-occlusion after thrombolysis

Re-occlusion of the culprit vessel remains the Achilles heel of thrombolytic therapy, and has been estimated to occur in approximately 20 per cent of cases where reperfusion was initially successful. However, in at least half of these, re-occlusion will be asymptomatic and detectable only with angiography. In a small proportion, re-occlusion will result in further pain and recurrent ST segment elevation, and these patients have an adverse prognosis. The optimal management of these cases remains unclear. Options should be discussed with a senior colleague, and include:

1. Repeat thrombolysis with rt-PA (since neutralizing antibodies may be present if patients have previously received streptokinase, and rt-PA is more likely to achieve rapid early reperfusion).

2. Referral for acute cardiac catheterization (especially when associated with haemodynamic compromise), resulting in:

   a. rescue PTCA

   b. surgical revascularization.

Key points

- Thrombolysis should be administered in all cases of acute MI presenting within 12 hours, in the presence of typical ECG changes and the absence of contraindications.

- Aim for a 'door-to-needle' time of 20 minutes or less.

- Streptokinase is the thrombolytic of choice in most circumstances, but rt-PA has beneficial effects in some subgroups.

- Aspirin should be given to all patients. Heparin is normally only given post rt-PA.

- Failure to reperfuse or re-occlusion after thrombolysis may be associated with a poor prognosis. These patients should be discussed with a senior colleague with a view to repeat thrombolysis or possibly rescue PTCA.

References

Cobbe, S. M. (1994). Thrombolysis in myocardial infarction. The earlier the better, but how late is too late? *Br. Med. J.*, **308**, 216–217.

Gershlick, A. H. and More, R. S. (1998). Treatment of myocardial infarction. *Br. Med. J.*, **316**, 280–284.

ISIS-3 collaborative group. (1993). ISIS-3: a randomized comparison of streptokinase vs. tissue plasminogen activator vs. anistreplase and of aspirin plus heparin vs. aspirin alone among 41 299 cases of suspected acute myocardial infarction. *Lancet*, **339**, 753–770.

Simoons, M. L., Boersma, E., Maas, A. C. P. *et al.* (1997). Management of myocardial infarction: the proper priorities. *Eur. Heart J.*, **18**, 896–899.

The GUSTO investigators. (1993). An international randomized trial comparing four thrombolytic strategies for acute myocardial infarction. *N. Engl. J. Med.*, **329**, 673–682.

The GUSTO angiographic investigators. (1993). The effects of tissue plasminogen activator, streptokinase, or both on coronary artery patency, ventricular function, and survival after acute myocardial infarction. *N. Engl. J. Med.*, **329**, 1615–1622.

The GUSTO investigators. (1997). A comparison of reteplase with alteplase for acute myocardial infarction. *N. Engl. J. Med.*, **337**, 1118–1123.

Update on thrombolytic agents: emerging options for AMI management. *Eur. Heart J.*, **18** (Suppl. F), F1–F35.

Ward, H. and Yudkin, J. S. (1995). Thrombolysis in patients with diabetes. *Br. Med. J.*, **310**, 3–4.

Weaver, W. D. (1996). The role of thrombolytic drugs in the management of myocardial infarction. *Eur. Heart J.*, **17** (Suppl. F), 9–15.

Yee, K. M. and Pringle, S. D. (1998). Failure of reperfusion following thrombolysis in acute myocardial infarction: a survey of current views and clinical practice. *Br. J. Cardiol.*, **5**, 35–40.

6

Beta-blocker and calcium antagonist therapy in acute myocardial infarction

Intravenous beta-blocker therapy in the early phase of acute myocardial infarction

Background

Early studies conducted in the 1970s and 1980s indicated that IV beta-blockers had a number of potentially advantageous effects in patients with acute MI. In the mid-1980s, the MIAMI and ISIS-1 study reported on the outcome in 25 000 patients randomized to IV beta-blockers or placebo. An overview of the published data indicates that, when used in selected patients in the course of acute MI in the pre-thrombolytic era, IV beta-blockers have the following attributes:

1. They are well tolerated, with over 95 per cent of appropriately selected patients able to receive full IV doses of beta-blockers without significant adverse effects.

2. They reduce early mortality (within the first 36 hours) by approximately 15 per cent. Subgroup analysis suggested that most of this mortality reduction was due to the prevention of cardiac rupture, and that mortality reduction was maximal in older patients with hypertension, a tachycardia or extensive infarction. Mortality reduction in low risk patients, who did not have any of these features, was minimal. The number of lives saved by IV beta-blockers is similar to that observed for early non-selective ACEI therapy in ISIS-4 and GISSI-3.

3. They limit infarct size and preserve left ventricular function.

4. They relieve ischaemic chest pain by reducing myocardial oxygen consumption.

5. They reduce the incidence of ventricular and supraventricular arrhythmias by blocking the deleterious effects of catecholamines and suppressing automaticity.

A number of studies have reported on the combined use of thrombolysis and IV beta-blockers. In the TIMI IIB study, almost 1500 patients were randomized to receive IV beta-blockade or deferred oral therapy starting on day six; IV beta-blockers were started shortly after thrombolytic therapy. The combination of thrombolytic therapy and IV beta-blockers was well tolerated, and was associated with a significant reduction in the incidence of early recurrent ischaemia, re-infarction, and cerebral haemorrhage. Recent data in large numbers of patients enrolled in GISSI-2, GUSTO, and a Swedish study also suggest that combined therapy improves outcome and is well tolerated.

Indications for IV beta-blocker therapy

Treatment with IV beta-blockers should be considered following the institution of thrombolytic therapy in all haemodynamically stable patients who present within 12 hours of the onset of symptoms of acute MI, with ST elevation in at least two leads, and who are free of contraindications. The groups of patients who will gain maximum benefit are:

1. Patients in whom thrombolytic therapy or PTCA are contraindicated or unavailable within 12 hours of the onset of symptoms
2. Patients with continuing ischaemic chest pain following thrombolytic therapy and IV analgesia
3. Patients at high risk of early complications (age > 65 years, extensive or anterior infarction, resting sinus tachycardia, past history of ischaemic heart disease, diabetes mellitus or hypertension)
4. Patients who are hypertensive (systolic BP > 160 mmHg), elderly or receive thrombolytic therapy relatively late, since these patients are at increased risk of early cardiac rupture.

Targeting IV beta-blocker therapy onto these four subgroups may help to maximize the gains from therapy, whilst limiting the number of patients who need to be treated. IV beta-blockers are preferable to nitrates for the control of peri-infarction hypertension (providing no contraindications are present), since they have additional beneficial effects on mortality.

Exclusion criteria for intravenous beta-blocker therapy

Patients are unsuitable for IV beta-blockers if:

1. The resting heart rate is below 50 bpm
2. Systolic blood pressure is below 100 mmHg
3. First, second or third degree heart block is present

4. Signs of left ventricular failure are present
5. Bronchospasm is present on admission, or the patient has a history of airways disease
6. Pre-treatment with a beta-blocker, diltiazem or verapamil has been given.

In patients with a marked resting tachycardia, it is important to exclude the presence of heart failure before administering IV beta-blockers.

Administration regime for intravenous atenolol

Atenolol is recommended for IV beta-blockade in acute MI, since its administration regime is relatively simple. Atenolol is given by slow IV injection, followed by oral atenolol, with the dose adjusted to slow the heart rate. The administration regime is as follows:

1. Give 5 mg atenolol by slow IV injection over five minutes. Stop if heart rate drops to 45 bpm or below, systolic blood pressure drops to 100 mmHg or below, the PR interval is prolonged to more than 0.26 s, or dyspnoea is aggravated.
2. If heart rate remains above 60 bpm ten minutes after initial IV bolus of atenolol, give a further IV injection of 2.5 mg, followed by a further 2.5 mg two minutes later (if necessary) to a maximum total dose of 10 mg over six minutes, observing the above cautions during each injection.
3. Ten minutes after the end of the IV injection, give 50 mg of oral atenolol if heart rate > 40 bpm.
4. Continue with long term oral atenolol 50–100 mg daily, unless a contra-indication develops.

Adverse effects of intravenous beta-blocker therapy

Adverse effects of IV beta-blocker therapy are very rare, occurring in less than 5 per cent of patients treated. Precipitation of heart failure and heart block are the commonest important side-effects, but are very rare in patients who have normal conduction and no evidence of heart failure. When these complications do occur they are easily reversible, and are not associated with an adverse effect on prognosis. Specific adverse effects are treated as follows:

1. Left ventricular failure should be treated by IV loop diuretics.
2. Symptomatic sinus bradycardia or complete heart block should be treated with IV atropine 0.6 mg, repeated as necessary. In rare cases, an infusion of a beta-agonist (such as dobutamine) or temporary pacing may be necessary.

3. Hypotension should initially be treated with a dobutamine infusion. If hypotension is severe and prolonged, and is thought to be related to beta-blocker therapy, an infusion of glucagon (50 mg/kg as an IV bolus followed by an infusion of 1–5 mg per hour) will reverse the effects of the beta-receptor blockade by increasing intracellular cAMP levels.

4. Bronchospasm may be precipitated in some susceptible individuals, and should be treated by withholding further doses of beta-blockers and treating the episode with nebulized beta-agonists.

Oral beta-blocker therapy in the convalescent phase of acute myocardial infarction

The use of oral beta-blockers in the convalescent phase of acute MI has been investigated in randomized controlled trials involving over 18 000 patients, which reported in the early 1980s. Meta-analysis of this data indicates that beta-blocker treatment is associated with a 25 per cent reduction in mortality due to re-infarction or sudden cardiac death during the years following an acute infarct. Beta-blockers have an antiarrhythmic effect, and subgroup analysis of the trials suggests that they reduce the occurrence of ventricular fibrillation. The reduced rate of re-infarction may relate to the drug's ability to protect atheromatous plaques from excessive haemodynamic stress effects, thereby reducing the rate of plaque rupture on subsequent MI.

All patients who do not have a contraindication should be commenced on an oral beta-blocker during the early (days 2–7) convalescent phase following an acute MI. Contraindications to oral beta-blocker therapy are present in around 20 per cent of post-infarct patients, and consist of:

1. Resting heart rate <50 bpm

2. Second or third degree heart block

3. A history of asthma, COPD or severe peripheral vascular disease.

Several different agents have been evaluated and shown to be effective. Since side-effects and compliance are problematic in some patients, a cardio-selective agent is preferable. Treatment should be started between days two and seven, with an agent such as metoprolol 50 mg bd, increased as necessary to obtain a resting heart rate of 50–60 bpm and continued indefinitely (a mortality benefit is still apparent up to six years after an infarction).

The maximum mortality benefit from beta-blocker therapy is obtained in higher risk patients, whose infarctions are complicated by arrhythmias or heart failure. These patients should initially be treated with appropriate antiarrhythmic and anti-failure therapy. Once their clinical condition is stabilized, a trial of beta-blocker therapy can be instituted. Treatment should be started with a low dose shorter acting agent such as metoprolol 25 mg bd, with the dose increased if tolerated.

Calcium antagonist therapy following acute myocardial infarction

A reduction in afterload, coronary vasodilatation and a reduction in intracellular calcium overload are potentially beneficial effects of calcium antagonists in patients with ischaemic heart disease.

Nifedipine has been extensively investigated in almost 10 000 patients (with the largest studies being TRENT, SPRINT-1, and SPRINT-2). In these trials there was a strong trend towards higher mortality in nifedipine-treated patients. This adverse effect of nifedipine may be related to its unopposed vasodilatation and reflex tachycardia.

Both diltiazem and verapamil have the additional effect of slowing the heart rate, which may improve their efficacy in post-infarction patients, and their use has been evaluated in three trials randomizing 8000 patients. In the DAVIT-1 trial, early use of verapamil had no beneficial effect and was associated with an increased risk of AV block or heart failure. In both the DAVIT-2 and MDPIT studies, verapamil and diltiazem started in the convalescent phase of acute MI were associated with a significant reduction in mortality and re-infarction rates, but only in the subgroup of patients with well preserved left ventricular function.

These studies indicate that calcium antagonists (particularly dihydropyridine agents) should be avoided in the acute phase of MI. In the convalescent phase, if a beta-blocker is contraindicated because of airways or peripheral vascular disease, and left ventricular function is good, verapamil 120 mg tds or diltiazem SR 90 mg bd are alternative agents for secondary prevention.

Key points

- IV beta-blockers are safe in selected patients, and reduce event rates in the first 36 hours after admission with acute MI.

- Combined therapy with thrombolytic agents and IV beta blockers is safe, well tolerated, and superior to the use of either agent alone.

- IV beta-blocker therapy exerts its maximum protective effect in high risk patients, who can be selected using simple clinical criteria.

- Oral beta-blockers started in the convalescent phase of acute MI are safe and effective in the secondary prevention of further cardiac events, particularly in patients who have arrhythmias or heart failure following an infarction.

- If a beta-blocker is contraindicated due to airways or peripheral vascular disease, calcium antagonist therapy with verapamil or diltiazem is an alternative for secondary prevention in patients with well preserved left ventricular function. Calcium antagonists (particularly dihydropyridine agents) should otherwise be avoided post-infarction.

References

Ball, S. G. (1998). Beta-blockers and antithrombotics for secondary prevention after myocardial infarction. *Eur. Heart J.*, **19**, 14–15.

Owen, A. (1998). Intravenous β blockade in acute myocardial infarction. Should be used in combination with thrombolysis. *Br. Med. J.*, **317**, 226–227.

Roberts, R., Rogers, W. J., Mueller, H. S., *et al.* (1991). Immediate versus deferred beta blockade following thrombolytic therapy in patients with acute MI. Results of the Thrombolysis in MI (TIMI) II-B Study. *Circulation*, **83**, 422–437.

Yusuf, S., Held, P. and Furberg, C. (1991). Update of effects of calcium antagonists in MI or angina in light of the second Danish Verapamil Infarction Trial (DAVIT-II) and other recent studies. *Am. J. Cardiol.*, **67**, 1295–1297.

Yusuf, S., Lessem, J., Jha, P., *et al.* (1993). Primary and secondary prevention of MI and strokes: an update of randomly allocated controlled trials. *J. Hypertens.*, **11** (Suppl. 4), 561–573.

7

Revascularization in acute myocardial infarction

Background

The introduction of coronary artery bypass grafting (CABG) in the late 1960s and percutaneous transluminal coronary angioplasty (PTCA) in the late 1970s have provided alternatives to medical therapy for the treatment of patients with ischaemic heart disease. A series of trials conducted in the last 20 years have clarified the roles of these two alternative forms of revascularization therapy in the treatment of patients with stable exertional angina. For patients with angina associated with left main stem disease, or with triple vessel disease and impaired left ventricular function, CABG will provide both symptomatic relief and prognostic benefit. In patients with single or double vessel disease, and those with triple vessel disease and good left ventricular function, CABG and PTCA offer no survival benefit compared with medical therapy. For patients with severe angina which is uncontrolled by medical therapy, either treatment modality is appropriate.

Treatment by PTCA is associated with a shorter initial hospital stay and lower initial costs, but with an increased need for intervention for recurrent symptoms associated with restenosis. Treatment by CABG is associated with a longer period of hospitalization and higher initial costs, but a low rate of reintervention in the first five years. The choice of treatment will depend on the precise coronary anatomy, and on patient preference. In the last 10 years, a series of trials have examined the roles of PTCA and CABG in the treatment of patients with acute MI, and this section will summarize their results.

Primary angioplasty

The theoretical basis for considering PTCA as the primary therapy for acute MI is based on the finding that treatment for infarction is only effective if it re-establishes early and adequate flow in the infarct-related artery. In recent trials, patients who achieve adequate reperfusion and a patent infarct-related artery have a mortality rate of less than two per cent, whilst those with inadequate flow have a mortality rate of 15–20 per cent. Currently, optimal thrombolytic therapy with accelerated rt-PA can achieve adequate flow in the infarct-related artery in only 54 per cent of patients 90 minutes after commencing treatment. Additionally, there is a small but unavoidable risk of death or disabling stroke due to intracerebral haemorrhage, and clinically significant re-occlusion of the infarct-related artery with recurrent ischaemia occurs in a proportion of patients following thrombolytic therapy. Because of these problems, a series of trials have recently compared primary angioplasty and thrombolytic therapy in the treatment of acute MI.

Ten randomized prospective trials have compared primary angioplasty with thrombolytic therapy in over 2500 patients. These studies show that PTCA can be carried out with a low complication rate, that adequate flow in the infarct-related artery can be established in over 90 per cent of patients, and that the risk of stroke following PTCA is very low. Additionally, PTCA is associated with a reduced risk of re-occlusion and recurrent ischaemia. The higher initial costs of PTCA may be offset by early discharge and a reduced need for reintervention. A meta-analysis of these 10 randomized studies suggests that primary PTCA may reduce mortality by about 30 per cent compared to thrombolytic therapy. Maximum mortality benefit is obtained in high risk patients. These studies were carried out by highly skilled operators in high volume institutions.

Recent retrospective studies of over 6000 patients treated with PTCA or thrombolytic therapy included results obtained by PTCA operators in less specialized, lower volume centres. This data suggests that primary PTCA in less specialized centres is less successful in achieving adequate flow in the infarct-related artery, and offers no survival advantage over a strategy of thrombolytic therapy followed by rescue PTCA for failed drug treatment.

Given the above data, it is clear that primary PTCA carried out by experienced operators is feasible, safe and effective in the treatment of acute MI. Since less than 10 per cent of the hospitals in Europe have facilities for PTCA, thrombolytic therapy will remain the best option for the early treatment of acute MI in most hospitals. Primary PTCA can be considered for patients for whom thrombolytic therapy is contraindicated, or in the 10 per cent of patients who present within six hours and can be classified as high risk on the basis of extensive ST segment change in association with adverse clinical features (two or more of the following: age > 70 years, anterior infarction, previous infarction, evidence of severe haemodynamic compromise or bundle branch block). Suitable patients admitted to hospitals that do not have facilities for PTCA should be discussed with a senior colleague. Recent data indicates that when primary PTCA is thought to be indicated because of contraindications to thrombolysis or high risk clinical features, transfer from peripheral hospitals to a PTCA centre is safe and there is no adverse effect on outcome if efforts are made to minimize delay in the centre.

Angioplasty following thrombolytic therapy

As discussed in the preceding section, thrombolytic therapy fails to restore adequate flow in a proportion of patients with acute MI. These patients have a relatively poor prognosis, with a high mortality rate and increased risk of heart failure. Failure to reperfuse with thrombolytic therapy is often associated with haemodynamic compromise, persistent chest pain and continuing ST segment elevation. Rescue PTCA compared with continued medical therapy in patients who fail to reperfuse has been evaluated in only a limited number of patients so far. Pooling the data on around 700 patients included in studies to date suggests that rescue PTCA can establish flow in the infarct-related artery in 80 per cent of patients, with a reduction in mortality to five per cent in some studies. If the clinical situation suggests failure to reperfuse 90 minutes after the administration of thrombolytic therapy, a senior colleague should be consulted because a rescue PTCA may improve outcome, particularly in patients with haemodynamic compromise (see Chapter 5).

Following successful thrombolytic therapy, patients are often left with a residual high grade stenosis which may cause further episodes of myocardial ischaemia. The strategy of carrying out routine angiography and PTCA in patients with suitable anatomy following thrombolytic therapy has been investigated in a series of important studies. In TAMI-I, ECSG, TIMI-IIA, TIMI-IIB and SWIFT, 4000 patients were randomized to early angiography and PTCA if the coronary anatomy was suitable, compared with a more conservative approach. Early non-selective intervention was not associated with beneficial effects on left ventricular function, death or recurrent ischaemia. On the basis of these trials, angiography and angioplasty should be reserved for patients who have continuing symptoms of ischaemia or an early positive exercise test.

Coronary artery bypass grafting

The results of elective CABG in patients with stable angina are excellent, with good symptom relief in the short to medium term, prognostic benefit in some subgroups, and operative mortality rates of less than one per cent. Following acute MI, CABG has only a limited role. Patients with uncontrolled angina post-infarction are at high risk of further infarction or death, and these patients should undergo angiography and PTCA if their coronary anatomy is suitable. If CABG is necessary, the perioperative mortality rate is around five per cent. The increased mortality may be related to the deleterious effect of cardiopulmonary bypass in a heart subjected to a recent infarction. Operative mortality rates are higher in women, diabetics, older patients and those with severe left ventricular impairment or previous CABG. If possible, surgery should be deferred for a few days to allow the haemodynamic state to stabilize and the effect of thrombolytic therapy to wear off.

Key points

- Primary PTCA is feasible and effective, and may produce superior results when carried out by highly skilled high volume operators, particularly in high risk patients.
- Facilities for primary PTCA are not available in most hospitals managing patients with acute MI.
- Thrombolytic therapy is widely available, easily and quickly administered, highly effective in improving survival, and does not require skilled personnel or catheterization laboratories.
- For most patients, thrombolytic therapy will remain the treatment of choice; for selected patients, primary PTCA should be considered, even if it is necessary to transfer the patient to another hospital for the procedure.
- Rescue PTCA may improve the prognosis in patients who fail to reperfuse or who develop haemodynamic compromise postinfarction.

References

Beat, K. J. and Fath-Ordoubadi, F. (1997). Angioplasty for the treatment of acute MI. *Heart*, **78** (Suppl. 2), 12–15.

Boersma, H., Van de Vlugt, M. J., Arnold, A. E. R., *et al.* (1996). Estimated gain in life expectancy. A simple tool to select optimal reperfusion treatment in individual patients with evolving MI. *Eur. Heart J.*, **17**, 64–75.

Brodie, B. R. (1997). When should patients with acute myocardial infarction be transferred for primary angioplasty? *Heart*, **78**, 327–328.

Every, N. R., Parsons, L. S., Hlatky, M., *et al*, for the MI Triage and Intervention Investigators. (1996). A comparison of thrombolytic therapy with primary coronary angioplasty for acute MI. *N. Engl. J. Med.*, **335**, 1253–1260.

Michels, K. B. and Yusuf, S. (1995). Does PTCA in acute myocardial infarction affect mortality and reinfarction rates? A quantitative overview (meta-analysis) of the randomized clinical trials. *Circulation*, **91**, 476–485.

8

Arrhythmias complicating acute myocardial infarction

Background

Tachyarrhythmias are very common in the first 24 hours following MI. Following admission to hospital, the majority (>90 per cent) of patients will have frequent ectopic beats, 20 per cent will have a life-threatening ventricular arrhythmia (usually within the first few hours of admission), and 15 per cent an episode of atrial fibrillation (AF). Tachyarrhythmias arise due to a combination of myocardial ischaemia and electrolyte abnormalities, leading to the development of re-entry circuits or enhanced automaticity. Tachyarrhythmias are more likely to occur in association with the sympathetic activation that often accompanies anterior infarction. The drug treatment of tachyarrhythmias is not uniformly effective, and frequently causes side-effects. The most serious side-effect is proarrhythmia, leading to the induction of further arrhythmias, which may lead to sudden cardiac death. Data from a series of trials published in the last decade provide some useful clinical guidelines for optimal therapy, and these will be referred to in the relevant sections of this chapter.

In the emergency treatment of tachyarrhythmias complicating acute MI, it is best to become familiar with a small number of drugs. The majority of post-infarction tachyarrhythmias can be effectively treated by lignocaine or amiodarone. If these agents are not effective, consult a senior colleague before using other unfamiliar drugs or combinations of agents, which may increase the risk of proarrhythmia.

Bradyarrhythmias occur in up to 30 per cent of post-infarction patients, with 5–10 per cent developing an episode of heart block. Bradyarrhythmias often arise in association with ischaemia or infarction of the specialized conduction system cells, and are more likely to occur in association with the vagal activation that often accompanies inferior infarction. When temporary pacing is required, the subclavian route should be avoided if thrombolytic therapy has been administered, as it will be difficult to ensure haemostasis if the subclavian artery is inadvertently punctured. Since the femoral vein is superficial and easy to compress, this is an appropriate access site in thrombolysed patients. The complication rate when inexperienced operators insert temporary pacemakers is high; where appropriate, bradyarrhythmias should be managed by observation or drug therapy, reserving pacemaker implantation for compromised or high risk patients.

When heart block occurs in a patient with inferior infarction, it is usually due to reversible ischaemia of the AV node. This usually recovers within a few hours or days, with a return to normal sinus rhythm. If complete heart block does develop, it is usually well tolerated. Since there is no damage to the conduction system in the ventricles, the secondary pacemaker that is responsible for ventricular activation will arise from a focus in the bundle of His. The escape rhythm generated from this secondary pacemaker will be conducted via the normal pathway to produce rapid ventricular activation, and the resultant rhythm will have a narrow QRS configuration. These secondary pacemakers in the bundle of His usually produce a stable reliable rhythm with a rate >40 bpm, which is often adequate to maintain the circulation with no compromise.

In contrast, when AV block develops in a patient with anterior infarction, it is often poorly tolerated and is associated with a high risk of early death. For AV block to occur in anterior infarction, extensive and widespread damage to the left ventricular myocardium and the interventricular septum must occur, and the patients often die from heart failure. In these patients, the conduction disturbance is related to infarction of the bundle of His within the interventricular septum. The secondary pacemaker that is responsible for ventricular activation will be situated outside the specialized conduction system in the surviving ventricular myocardium. The escape rhythm generated by this type of secondary pacemaker will often have an unreliable rate of <40 bpm (since the inherent automaticity of cells outside the specialized conduction system is usually low), and will have a broad QRS configuration as ventricular activation will be slow. This slow rate will be poorly tolerated in a patient with extensive ventricular damage, and episodes of unpredictable ventricular asystole often occur. When AV block occurs following acute anterior infarction, temporary pacing is usually required. If the patient survives the acute episode, the AV block is often persistent or recurrent, and a permanent pacemaker may be required.

In extensive anterior infarction with involvement of the septum, ischaemic damage to the bundle of His may lead to left or right bundle branch block on the surface ECG. The development of left bundle branch block usually indicates that extensive myocardial necrosis has occurred, with associated significant left ventricular dysfunction and a poor prognosis. Right bundle branch block can occur with less extensive infarction, as can involvement of only the anterior fasicle of the left bundle, leading to left axis deviation. Patients who develop left bundle branch block in combination with a long PR interval, or the combination of right bundle branch block, left axis deviation and a long PR interval, have suffered extensive damage to their conduction system and should be discussed with a senior colleague, as prophylactic temporary pacing may be indicated to avert the need for pacemaker insertion in a compromised patient if sudden complete heart block with a slow escape rhythm develops.

The remainder of this chapter will discuss the treatment of specific arrhythmias.

Tachyarrythmias

Supraventricular and ventricular ectopic beats

Supraventricular ectopic beats are due to the premature discharge of an ectopic focus in the atria or the AV junction. Since ventricular activation occurs via the normal conduction system, supraventricular ectopics are characterized by a QRS complex of normal morphology, which occurs prematurely and may be preceded by an abnormal P-wave (Figure 8.1). Ventricular ectopic beats arise due to the premature discharge of an ectopic focus in the ventricular myocardium. Ventricular activation occurs slowly, producing a QRS complex with a broad configuration (Figure 8.2). Supraventricular and ventricular ectopics are very common after acute MI, and there is no evidence that pharmacological suppression of ectopic activity prevents the occurrence of life-threatening ventricular arrhythmias or improves prognosis. When frequent ectopics occur:

1. Ensure that pain relief is adequate – if continuing ischaemic pain is present, consider the use of IV beta-blockade or further diamorphine

2. Look for and treat heart failure if present

3. Check electrolytes, and give supplements if potassium <4.0 mmol/l (Chapter 24). Consider giving intravenous magnesium if the patient has been on long-term diuretic therapy prior to admission.

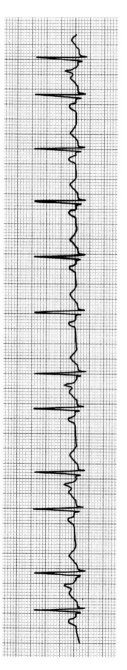

Figure 8.1 Supraventricular ectopic beats. Each ectopic occurs prematurely, and is preceded by a morphologically abnormal P-wave.

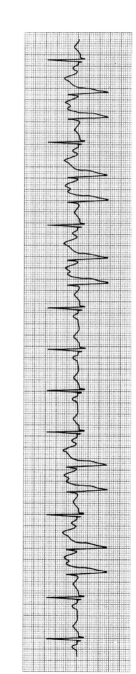

Figure 8.2 Ventricular ectopic beats. Each ectopic is premature and has a broad QRS morphology.

Sinus tachycardia

Sinus tachycardia is common after an acute MI, and is often associated with extensive anterior infarction, sympathetic activation and an adverse prognosis. In sinus tachycardia, each QRS complex is preceded by a normal P-wave, the QRS complexes are of normal morphology, and the rate is normally less than 140 bpm. If sinus tachycardia is persistent and excessive, it may cause extension of myocardial necrosis by increasing oxygen consumption. If sinus tachycardia is persistent:

1. Ensure analgesia is adequate
2. Look for and treat heart failure
3. Consider IV beta-blockade if there are no contraindications.

Prolonged sinus tachycardia is most likely to occur in a patient with extensive infarction and major left ventricular impairment, and it is more likely that additional analgesia or heart failure treatment will be required, rather than a beta-blocker.

Atrial fibrillation

Atrial fibrillation is the most common supraventricular arrhythmia after acute MI. It is frequently associated with extensive anterior infarction, and implies an adverse prognosis. Post-infarction AF is due to atrial infarction or stretch generating multiple and changing micro re-entry circuits within the atrium. Chaotic atrial activity is intermittently conducted via the AV node to depolarize the ventricles. Characteristic ECG features of AF are an irregular baseline due to fibrillation waves (often best seen in V1) with completely irregular ventricular activity (Figure 8.3). The QRS complexes are narrow, unless bundle branch block is also present. Treatment of post-infarction AF depends on the ventricular rate and associated features:

1. If the ventricular rate is rapid (>200 bpm), systolic BP is low (<90 mmHg) or the arrhythmia is associated with chest pain, heart failure or impaired consciousness, DC cardioversion is the treatment of choice.
2. Many episodes of post-infarction AF are short-lived (50 per cent last less than 30 minutes) and well tolerated. If AF occurs with a rate of <110 bpm, systolic blood pressure is maintained above 90 mmHg and there are no associated symptoms, no treatment is necessary initially.
3. If AF persists for more than 30 minutes, has a rate consistently >110 bpm, is associated with a fall in systolic BP or with rate-related symptoms, drug treatment is indicated.

Digoxin is relatively ineffective at slowing ventricular rate in post-

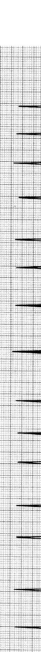

Figure 8.3 Atrial fibrillation. There is a completely irregular ventricular rhythm, with erratic atrial fibrillatory activity visible between the QRS complexes.

infarction patients with high levels of circulating catecholamines, may increase the propensity for life-threatening ventricular arrhythmias, and is ineffective at restoring sinus rhythm. Intravenous amiodarone rapidly slows the ventricular rate, converts 75 per cent of patients back to sinus rhythm within four hours, and is our first line drug therapy for persistent post-infarction AF. Intravenous amiodarone infusions can be administered via a peripheral line, provided that a large calibre vein is used, and the amiodarone solution is < 2mg/ml. If a prolonged or high concentration infusion is required, administration via a central vein will be necessary to avoid thrombophlebitis. It is important to follow the initial intravenous bolus with a 24 hour infusion, since there is otherwise a high risk of recurrent episodes of AF during this period. If AF persists after the first 24 hours, anticoagulation and planned cardioversion should be considered. Other atrial arrhythmias are uncommon in post-infarction patients, and their management is dealt with in detail in Chapter 18.

Ventricular tachyarrhythmias

Ventricular tachyarrhythmias are common following acute MI. The prognostic significance depends on the type of arrhythmia and on its timing in relation to the infarction:

1. Ventricular tachyarrhythmias which occur within the first 24 hours of infarction are related to re-entry in ischaemic myocardium, are not likely to recur, and are not associated with a bad prognosis.

2. Ventricular tachyarrhythmias which occur after the first 24 hours are usually related to re-entry mechanisms associated with scar tissue at the interface between infarcted and normal myocardium. Late ventricular tachyarrhythmias are usually associated with large infarctions, and are more likely to recur.

In general, early ventricular tachyarrhythmias do not require long-term drug therapy. Late ventricular tachyarrhythmias frequently recur and cause sudden cardiac death. Empirical antiarrhythmic drug therapy is not likely to be successful in these patients, and they should all be assessed by an electrophysiologist, as EP-guided drug therapy or AICD implantation improve their prognosis. Some patients are not suitable for AICD implantation or EP studies because of other medical problems. The CAST study confirmed that Class-1 antiarrhythmic agents have an adverse effect on mortality following a recent infarction, and should be avoided. A recent meta-analysis of 6500 patients enrolled in randomized placebo-controlled trials of amiodarone suggests that this drug reduces total mortality by 13 per cent, and sudden death by 29 per cent. If empirical drug therapy is necessary, amiodarone is the agent of choice.

Non-sustained ventricular arrhythmias

Non-sustained ventricular arrhythmias (frequent ectopic beats, couplets, triplets and bursts of consecutive ectopic beats lasting less than 10 seconds) are very common after acute MI, and are usually asymptomatic. Frequent non-sustained ventricular arrhythmias are a poor prognostic feature, and are associated with an increased mortality rate of 15 per cent in the first year after infarction. Treatment of asymptomatic non-sustained ventricular arrhythmias with Class-1 antiarrhythmic drugs following MI was investigated in the placebo-controlled CAST study. Despite suppression of antiarrhythmias, mortality was increased by drug therapy. The results of CAST indicate that, despite the poor prognosis associated with the occurrence of frequent arrhythmias, they should not be treated with Class-1 antiarrhythmic drugs.

Sustained monomorphic ventricular tachycardia

In post-infarction patients, monomorphic ventricular tachycardia (VT) presents as a regular, broad complex tachycardia with a stable QRS configuration and a rate greater than 120 bpm (Figure 8.4), and should be treated as a medical emergency, as the tachycardia may degenerate to VF with cardiac arrest. A relatively slow monomorphic VT in a patient with reasonable left ventricular function may be tolerated without major haemodynamic compromise, whilst a rapid monomorphic VT in a patient with significant LV impairment will be poorly tolerated and associated with haemodynamic collapse. The treatment of sustained monomorphic VT depends on the degree of haemodynamic impairment that occurs:

1. If systolic BP <90 mmHg or the patient has chest pain or heart failure related to the tachycardia, DC cardioversion is the treatment of choice. If consciousness is lost with the onset of VT, administer the shock immediately. If the patient remains conscious despite haemodynamic compromise, sedate with 2–10 mg of IV midazolam prior to cardioversion.

2. If systolic BP >90 mmHg and the patient is not distressed or poorly perfused, initial treatment should be with lignocaine 50 mg IV over two minutes, repeated every five minutes if the arrhythmia does not terminate, to a maximum dose of 200 mg. Lignocaine is preferable to other Class-1 agents since its vasoconstrictor properties limit the occurrence of drug-induced hypotension, and its initial short half-life enables

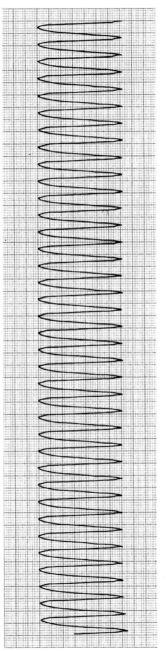

Figure 8.4 Sustained monomorphic VT. Rapid regular broad complex tachycardia (rate 210 bpm).

other antiarrhythmic agents to be administered if it is initially ineffective without an excessive risk of drug interaction. It is, however, effective in terminating VT in only 20 per cent of patients.

3. If the lignocaine bolus terminates the VT, commence an infusion of 500 mg of lignocaine in 500 ml of 5% dextrose at an infusion rate of 4 mg/minute for 30 minutes, 2 mg/minute for two hours and 1 mg/minute for 24 hours. Since lignocaine is metabolized in the liver, reduce the infusion rate in patients with liver disease or impaired hepatic perfusion due to heart failure. Check electrolytes, blood gases and look for clinical evidence of heart failure. Treat failure with diuretics or nitrates, and give oxygen if hypoxia is present. If serum potassium is less than 4.0 mmol/l, give potassium supplements IV as detailed in Chapter 24.

4. If VT recurs despite the lignocaine infusion, give a further bolus of 100 mg lignocaine and increase the infusion rate to 2 mg/minute for one hour, and give IV magnesium as detailed in Chapter 24.

5. If the VT is not terminated by the initial bolus of 200 mg of lignocaine, or recurs despite an infusion and further boluses of lignocaine plus administration of potassium and magnesium and the patient remains haemodynamically stable, amiodarone has demonstrated the ability to suppress VT resistent to Class-1 agents in 90 per cent of patients. Discontinue treatment with lignocaine and give amiodarone IV as detailed in Chapter 24.

6. *If VT persists and the patient deteriorates haemodynamically during lignocaine or amiodarone administration, carry out immediate DC cardioversion.* If both lignocaine and amiodarone fail to terminate the VT, further drug therapy is contraindicated, as administration of multiple antiarrhythmics will increase the risk of adverse effects. Continue the amiodarone infusion and carry out DC cardioversion. Consult a senior colleague regarding further therapy.

7. If frequent episodes of VT recur despite amiodarone infusion, temporary overdrive pacing may be effective in terminating episodes. Insert a pacing lead into the right ventricle. When VT occurs, pace at a rate 20 per cent faster than the VT for 10 seconds, then abruptly discontinue the pacing. If the pacing therapy is successful, sinus rhythm will return. Rapid VT or VF may be precipitated by overdrive pacing, requiring immediate DC cardioversion.

Polymorphic ventricular tachycardia

In post-infarction patients, polymorphic VT presents as a rapid (rate >200 bpm) ventricular arrhythmia with continuously varying QRS morphology. Polymorphic VT is usually poorly tolerated and rapidly progresses to VF and cardiac arrest. Since cardiac arrest invariably accompanies sustained polymorphic VT, immediate DC cardioversion is required. Following DC cardioversion:

1. Check the 12 lead ECG and measure the longest QT interval. If this is less than 0.42 seconds, commence a lignocaine infusion.
2. Look for and correct hypokalaemia, hypoxia and heart failure.
3. Give magnesium IV (see Chapter 24).

Post-infarction polymorphic VT is rarely associated with QT prolongation unless the patient has been previously treated with antiarrhythmic drugs or with other drugs known to prolong the QT interval, such as phenothiazines, tricyclics, antihistamines or erythromycin. If drug therapy has induced QT prolongation complicated by polymorphic VT, withdraw the responsible agent, correct hypokalaemia, give magnesium, institute temporary pacing at a rate of at least 100 bpm to shorten the QT interval, and continue with the rapid ventricular pacing until the QT interval normalizes.

Ventricular fibrillation

In post-infarction patients, VF presents with rapid chaotic electrical activity leading to loss of co-ordinated ventricular contraction and cardiorespiratory arrest. VF is a common cause of death in patients with acute MI. Most episodes occur within four hours of the onset of symptoms. In hospitalized patients with no evidence of heart failure, resuscitation from VF and long-term survival are good. When VF occurs in hospitalized patients with haemodynamic compromise, only 20 per cent of patients survive to leave hospital. Prophylactic lignocaine does not improve survival in infarct patients, and is not recommended. Correction of hypokalaemia halves the risk of VF, and supplements should be given to all patients with a potassium concentration of < 4.0 mmol/l. When VF occurs, the treatment is immediate defibrillation and cardiopulmonary resuscitation, as detailed in Chapter 9.

Idioventricular rhythm

Idioventricular rhythm presents as a regular broad complex tachycardia with a stable QRS configuration and a rate of less than 120 bpm (Figure 8.5), and occurs in 20 per cent of patients in the early post-infarction phase. Idioventricular rhythm often occurs in association with reperfusion following thrombolytic therapy, is rarely associated with any haemodynamic impairment and does not usually degenerate into life-threatening ventricular tachyarrhythmias. Since the arrhythmia is well

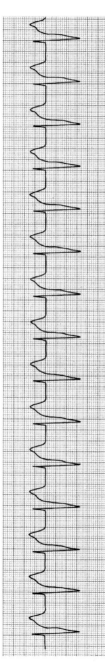

Figure 8.5 Idioventricular rhythm. Regular broad complex tachycardia (rate 75 bpm).

tolerated and not associated with progression to more serious tachy-carrhythmias, no treatment is necessary.

Bradyarrhythmias

Sinus bradycardia and sinus arrest

Sinus bradycardia is common in the early stages of acute infarction, but rarely requires treatment. The ECG will show normal QRS complexes preceded by a normal P-wave, with a rate of <60 bpm (Figure 8.6). Occasionally, intermittent sinus arrest occurs in inferior infarction due to ischaemia of the sinus node or activation of cardiac vagal reflexes during reperfusion of an occluded right coronary artery. If the heart rate is persistently below 45 bpm due to sinus bradycardia or periods of sinus arrest, in association with symptoms or clinical signs of reduced cardiac output, a bolus of atropine 0.6 mg intravenously will increase the sinus rate. If necessary, the dose of atropine can be repeated. If symptomatic sinus bradycardia is persistent despite repeated atropine, it may be necessary to consider temporary pacing.

First degree heart block

First degree heart block manifests as prolongation of the PR interval, and is common in inferior infarction (Figure 8.7). Forty per cent of patients with inferior infarction and first degree heart block progress to self-terminating and well tolerated episodes of Wenckebach or complete heart block. In anterior infarction, first degree heart block is usually a sign of extensive myocardial necrosis with septal involvement. First degree heart block requires no specific treatment (other than avoiding drugs such as beta-blockers, which prolong AV conduction), but the patient requires close monitoring (particularly in anterior infarcts) for progression to higher degrees of block or other complications.

Mobitz type I second degree heart block (Wenckebach phenomenon)

Mobitz type I block manifests as increasing prolongation of the PR interval until a QRS complex is dropped as a result of complete failure of AV nodal conduction, and is usually the result of AV nodal ischaemia in inferior infarction (Figure 8.8). If complete heart block develops, it is usually associated with a narrow complex escape rhythm which is well tolerated. Apart from avoiding AV nodal blocking drugs, no active treatment other than close observation of the patient is usually required.

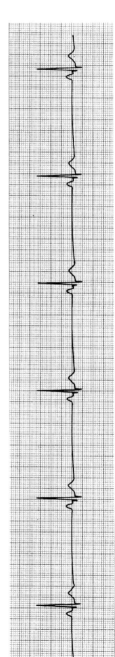

Figure 8.6 Sinus bradycardia. Each QRS complex is preceded by a morphologically normal P-wave. Heart rate is slow (30 bpm).

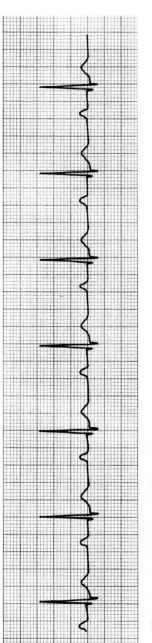

Figure 8.7 First degree heart block. PR interval is 0.32 seconds.

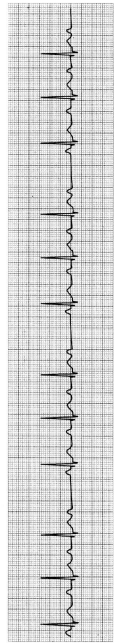

Figure 8.8 Mobitz type I block. There is a progressive increase in PR interval with each successive sinus beat, until complete failure of AV nodal conduction occurs. The sequence is then repeated.

Mobitz type II second degree block

Mobitz type II block manifests itself as sudden unpredictable failure of AV nodal conduction, resulting in a dropped beat with no preceding change in the PR interval (Figure 8.9). Mobitz type II block is usually associated with septal involvement in extensive anterior infarction leading to ischaemic damage to the bundle of His, and often co-exists with bundle branch block. Mobitz type II block frequently progresses to poorly tolerated complete heart block with a slow and unreliable broad complex escape rhythm. Patients with anterior infarction who develop Mobitz type II block have a poor prognosis. When Mobitz type II block occurs, consult a senior colleague, as prophylactic temporary pacing may be indicated to avert the need for pacemaker insertion in a compromised patient if sudden complete heart block with a slow escape rhythm develops.

Third degree (complete) heart block

Complete heart block presents with complete dissociation between atrial and ventricular activity (Figure 8.10). The pathophysiology and recommended treatment depend on the site of infarction associated with the heart block.

In inferior infarction, patients usually progress through first degree and Wenckebach block to well tolerated complete heart block with a narrow complex escape rhythm. If the blood pressure is well maintained and the patient is asymptomatic, no treatment is necessary. If the ventricular rate falls below 40 bpm, pauses of >3 seconds occur, the systolic BP falls below 90 mmHg or rate-related symptoms develop:

1. Give atropine 0.6 mg intravenously, repeated as necessary.
2. If symptomatic complete heart block persists despite atropine, insert a temporary pacing wire.

Normal AV nodal conduction usually returns within 48 hours, a permanent pacemaker is not required, and prognosis after discharge from hospital is good.

In patients with anterior infarction, complete heart block often occurs suddenly, particularly in patients who develop left bundle branch block or have a period of Mobitz type II block. The escape rhythm is broad complex and slow, often associated with severe haemodynamic compromise in a patient with extensive infarction and major left ventricular impairment. Temporary pacing is always required to maintain an adequate rate. High grade AV block often persists, necessitating perma-

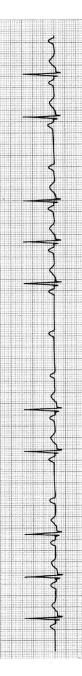

Figure 8.9 Mobitz type II block. The PR interval in conducted beats is normal. Sudden failure of AV nodal conduction occurs unpredictably, resulting in non-conducted P-waves which are not followed by a QRS complex.

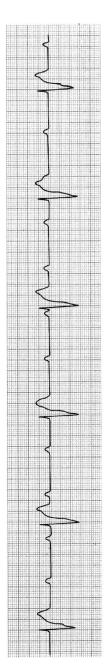

Figure 8.10 Third degree (complete) heart block. P-waves and QRS complexes are completely dissociated. Ventricular rhythm is broad complex and slow (30 bpm).

nent pacemaker implantation. A large proportion (80 per cent) of patients who develop complete heart block following anterior infarction die, often from pump failure due to ventricular damage.

Key points

- Arrhythmias are very common after acute infarction. The majority of patients have frequent ectopics. Tachyarrhythmias are more common after anterior infarction, bradyarrhythmias after inferior infarction.

- Sinus tachycardia is often associated with untreated heart failure or residual ischaemic chest pain.

- Frequent ectopic beats and non-sustained VT do not require drug therapy.

- Many episodes of AF are well tolerated and resolve spontaneously. If drug treatment is necessary, intravenous amiodarone is our first choice therapy.

- Late ventricular arrhythmias are usually associated with large infarctions, have a tendency to recur, and require expert assessment by a clinical electrophysiologist to reduce the high risk of sudden cardiac death.

- Avoid polypharmacy in the drug treatment of VT. Lignocaine and amiodarone are the first and second line drugs of choice.

- Bradyarrhythmias complicating inferior infarction are usually well tolerated and do not imply a poor prognosis. Bradyarrhythmias complicating anterior infarction are associated with extensive infarction, are poorly tolerated, and imply a poor prognosis.

References

Amiodarone Trials Meta-analysis Investigators. (1997). Effect of prophylactic amiodarone on mortality after acute myocardial infarction and in congestive heart failure: meta-analysis of individual data 6500 patients in randomized trials. *Lancet*, **350**, 1417–1421.

Chamberlain, D. (1997). Periarrest arrhythmias. *Br. J. Anaesth.*, **79**, 198–202.

Cowan, J. C., Gardiner, P., Reid, D. S., *et al.* (1986). Amiodarone in the management of atrial fibrillation complicating MI. *Brit. J. Clin. Pract.*, **40**, 155–161.

Echt, D. S., Liebson, P. R., Mitchell, B., *et al.* (1991). Mortality and morbidity in patients receiving encainide, flecainide or placebo – The Cardiac Arrhythmia Suppression Trial. *N. Engl. J. Med.*, **324**, 781–788.

Kowey, P. R., Marinchak, R. A., Rials, S. J., *et al.* Intravenous amiodarone. *J. Am. Coll. Cardiol.*, **29**, 1190–1198.

Lawrie, D. M., Higgins, M. R., Godman, M. J., *et al.* (1968). Ventricular fibrillation complicating acute MI. *Lancet*, **2**, 523–528.

Rankin, A. C. and Cobbe, S. M. (1993). Broad-complex tachycardias. *Prescribers Journal*, **33**, 138–146.

The Task Force on the Management of Acute MI of the European Society of Cardiology. (1996). Acute MI, pre-hospital and in-hospital management. *Eur. Heart J.*, **17**, 43–63.

9

Resuscitation

Background

Patients admitted to the coronary care unit with unstable cardiovascular disease are at high risk of life-threatening arrhythmias and cardiac arrest, and all staff involved in patient care should be trained to a high level in cardiopulmonary resuscitation. Although data from randomized controlled trials is limited, techniques for cardiopulmonary resuscitation have been standardized in recent years, and the guidelines in this chapter are based on those published by the European Resuscitation Council in 1998. This chapter aims to provide concise contemporary guidelines for the emergency treatment of ventricular fibrillation, asystole and electromechanical dissociation. Life support by means of ventilation and external cardiac massage are not covered in this chapter. Medical and nursing staff with responsibility for managing patients on coronary care units should attend courses which teach these practical aspects of cardiopulmonary resuscitation, and aim for recertification on a regular basis to ensure that they remain up to date.

Patients who suffer cardiac arrest in hospital are usually attached to rhythm monitors, and the underlying rhythm can usually be rapidly identified. Patients who develop VF without evidence of severe heart failure are usually successfully resuscitated and have a good long-term prognosis. Patients who develop VF or asystole complicating severe heart failure have a poor prognosis. Resuscitation is often unsuccessful; even when it is initially successful, recurrent arrhythmias are common, as is death due to intractable heart failure, and the long-term prognosis is poor. When electromechanical dissociation occurs in a patient with a recent MI, it is usually due to rupture of the left ventricular free wall, and resuscitation is rarely successful.

Ventricular fibrillation

This is recognized on the cardiac monitor by the presence of chaotic fibrillation waves, due to wandering of cardiac electrical activity along continuously changing pathways (Figure 9.1). Check for absence of pulse. A precordial thump administered to the lower sternum may revert the patient to sinus rhythm. If this fails, proceed to defibrillation as soon as possible.

1. Initial treatment is a 200 J shock. If VF persists after the first shock, give a further 200 J shock, followed by a 360 J shock if necessary. The shocks should be given as close together as possible, without intervals for CPR. Patients who do not respond to one of these first three shocks have a low probability of survival.

2. If VF still persists, intubate the patient and give 1 mg of adrenaline IV (10 ml of a 1:10 000 solution). Institute basic life support with 10 CPR sequences of 5:1 compression/ventilation, and repeat the 360 J shock three times if necessary. Look for and treat aggravating factors such as electrolyte disturbance, hypothermia or drug overdose.

3. If VF still persists, continue CPR, interrupting for a further three shocks of 360 J after each minute. Give 1 mg of adrenaline IV every three minutes.

4. If VF still persists, give 50 ml of 8.4% bicarbonate IV and 100 mg of lignocaine IV followed by 10 CPR sequences, then repeat 3×360 J shocks.

5. If VF persists, give bretylium 5–10 mg/kg IV. This drug may take up to 30 minutes to exert its full antifibrillatory effect, and resuscitation should therefore continue for at least this time period once it has been administered.

6. If VF persists, consider:
   a. Different paddle positions or a different defibrillator
   b. Magnesium IV (see Chapter 24 for regime).

After successful resuscitation from VF, commence IV treatment with an antiarrhythmic agent (lignocaine or amiodarone) or with magnesium for the next 24 hours to suppress recurrent ventricular arrhythmias. The question of long-term antiarrhythmic therapy and the indications for electrophysiological testing are dealt with in Chapter 8.

Asystole

This is recognized by the total absence of any ventricular electrical activity on the cardiac monitor (Figure 9.2). Check that the monitor is working by tapping a chest electrode and looking for artefacts. If any

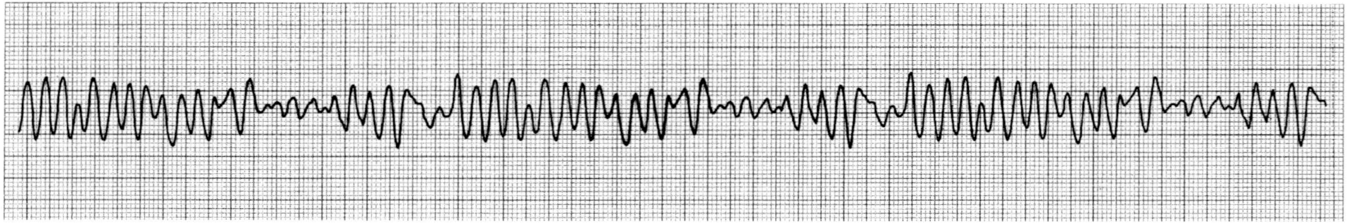

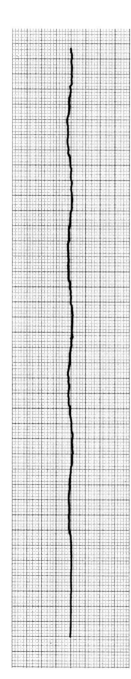

Figure 9.1 Chaotic ventricular electrical activity in VF.

Figure 9.2 Absent myocardial electrical activity in asystole.

doubt exists in your mind that the trace is unreliable and that undetected VF may be present, initial treatment should be with a precordial thump and $3 \times DC$ shocks (200 J, 200 J, then 360 J). If these are unsuccessful, intubate and proceed as detailed below:

1. Give adrenaline 1 mg IV, followed by 10 CPR sequences of 5:1 compression/ventilation.

2. If asystole persists, give atropine 3 mg IV (once only). If no electrical activity is evident, give a further 1 mg adrenaline followed by 10 CPR sequences.

3. If asystole persists with no electrical activity, give a further 1 mg of adrenaline IV and repeat 10 CPR sequences.

4. If asystole persists with no electrical activity, give 5 mg adrenaline IV followed by 10 CPR sequences. If there is no response to this, successful resuscitation is unlikely. If electrical activity is evident after the above manoeuvres, consider external cardiac pacing. Pacing will be useful only if the heart has recovered at least some electrical activity.

Electromechanical dissociation (EMD)

This is recognized by the presence of ventricular complexes with an adequate rate on the monitor, with no cardiac output. The commonest cause of sudden, unexpected development of electromechanical dissociation following acute MI is rupture of the ventricular free wall. Successful resuscitation in this situation is very rare. Other important causes to consider are:

1. Pneumothorax – have a high index of suspicion in patients with chronic airways disease or those in whom a central line has been recently inserted.

2. Pulmonary embolism – particularly in bedbound or postoperative patients.

3. Hypovolaemia – is there any obvious cause of blood loss?

4. Drug toxicity – particularly in patients with a history of drug overdose.

5. Cardiac tamponade – this should be suspected in patients who are at risk (chronic renal failure, connective tissue disorder, neoplastic disease, aortic dissection), and must be ruled out in patients with EMD after a stab wound or other chest trauma.

6. Hypothermia – prolonged resuscitation should be considered in such patients, since full recovery without neurological sequelae is possible (particularly in children).

Having instituted basic life support, ascertained the presence of electromechanical dissociation and instituted any specific therapy necessary for the conditions above, intubate the patient and continue CPR. Further treatment consists of:

1. Give adrenaline 1 mg every three minutes
2. If EMD still persists, give 50 ml of 8.4% sodium bicarbonate and 5 mg of adrenaline IV followed by 10 CPR sequences.

If EMD persists and no readily reversible cause is apparent, successful resuscitation is unlikely. Resuscitation from EMD consists of finding and treating the cause, if possible.

Post-resuscitation care

Immediately after an arrest, check blood gases, electrolytes and an ECG, and treat any problems; e.g.:

1. Maintain potassium above 4.0 mmol/l (see Chapter 24). If potassium is above 6.0, give 10 ml of 10% calcium chloride IV over 5 minutes, and follow this with 50 ml of 50% dextrose and 10 units of short acting insulin to stabilize the myocardium and correct the hyperkalaemia. Recheck potassium at regular intervals to ensure optimal plasma level is maintained.
2. Control hyperglycaemia with a sliding scale insulin infusion (avoiding hypoglycaemia, which may exacerbate neurological injury) as detailed in Chapter 24.
3. Hypoxia is usually present, so give oxygen. Monitor the efficiency of supplemental oxygen using pulse oximetry, increasing the oxygen concentration to maintain saturation > 93 per cent. If persistent acidosis is present, consider the use of bicarbonate given in 25 ml boluses to maintain the serum pH at 7.3–7.5.
4. Arrange a portable CXR, and treat any pneumothorax.
5. Consider lignocaine, amiodarone or magnesium infusions where indicated.
6. Treat left ventricular failure if present. Look for and treat any persistent cardiac ischaemia that may have precipitated the cardiac arrest.
7. Treat hypotension if present. If hypotension persists, consider a pulmonary artery catheter to guide optimal fluid and inotropic therapy.
8. Monitor urine output and use dopamine (2.5–5.0 mcg/kg/min) as detailed in Chapter 24 if output is less than 30 ml/hour for two consecutive hours.

Following a successful resuscitation, most patients will regain consciousness rapidly. Hypoxia must be avoided after resuscitation, and assisted ventilation should be used if there is a reasonable chance of recovery. If the patient remains unconscious and dependent on assisted ventilation, either transfer to the general intensive care unit or seek advice from an anaesthetics colleague on ventilatory management. The decision to withdraw ventilatory support is probably best made by a senior colleague, and advice should be sought in this situation.

Decision making

No hard and fast rules exist. If asystole or EMD persists after 20 minutes of resuscitation in a normothermic adult without drug toxicity, then success is unlikely and the attempt should probably be abandoned. If VF persists at this point, the situation is still potentially reversible, and it may be worth persisting with attempts at resuscitation. When hypothermia is present, attempts to revive the patient should continue for longer, probably until core temperature is above 36°C and arterial pH and potassium are normal, since full recovery has been documented after prolonged resuscitation in such patients. Do not use pupillary dilatation as your only reason for stopping resuscitation, as this can be drug induced. Do not be overconcerned about long-term brain damage. Few patients with brain damage secondary to cardiac arrest from heart disease survive long-term.

Key points

- Successful resuscitation from witnessed ventricular arrhythmias in a patient with well preserved left ventricular function is the norm. Resuscitation from ventricular arrhythmias in a patient with severe impairment of left ventricular function, asystole, electromechanical dissociation or unwitnessed cardiac arrest is less common.

- Remember to give repeated boluses of adrenaline, usually every three minutes.

- In electromechanical dissociation, look for treatable causes before abandoning resuscitation.

- Careful post-resuscitation care is essential to maximize the chances of a full recovery.

References

Advanced Life Support Working Group of the European Resuscitation Council (1998). The European Resuscitation Council Guidelines for adult advanced life support. *Br. Med. J.*, **316**, 1863–1869.

Bacauer, M. B. (1986). Treatment of ventricular fibrillation and other acute arrhythmias with bretylium tosylate. *Am. J. Cardiol.*, **21**, 530.

Ballew, K. A. (1997). Cardiopulmonary resuscitation. *Br. Med. J.*, **314**, 1462–1465.

Nolan, J. (1998). 1998 European guidelines on resuscitation. *Br. Med. J.*, **316**, 1844–1845.

Wenger, T. L., Lederman, S., Startmer, F., *et al.* (1984). A method for quantitating antifibrillatory effects of drugs after coronary reperfusion in dogs: improved outcome with bretylium. *Circulation*, **69**, 142–148.

10   Acute pulmonary oedema

Background

Acute pulmonary oedema is a life-threatening emergency, and should be treated immediately. However, it is important to realize that there are many different aetiologies. The commonest cause is left ventricular failure (LVF) in the setting of an acute MI. Other causes of pulmonary oedema in the absence of a failing left ventricle include:

1. Mitral valve disease
2. Cardiac arrhythmias
3. Cardiac tamponade
4. Septicaemia
5. Acute renal failure
6. Adult respiratory distress syndrome (ARDS).

These conditions need to be actively excluded and/or specifically treated.

The development of LVF is common after extensive MI. Its occurrence is an adverse prognostic feature, with close correlation between the degree of LVF and mortality. This fact has been recognized for many years, and was demonstrated by Killip's classification in 1967 (Table 10.1) (Killip and Kimball, 1967). Despite modern therapy for acute MI, analysis of data in the GUSTO trial in 1993 showed that mortality remains high in patients with heart failure following infarction.

The diagnosis of LVF should never be made on the basis of basal crepitations alone; these are often due to co-existent lung disease (e.g. small airways disease, pulmonary fibrosis, concurrent infection). The diagnosis is probable when two or more of the following are present:

1. A prominent third heart sound (S3) is audible, with or without sinus tachycardia
2. Basal crackles, which do not clear with coughing

Table 10.1 Killip classification of severity of infarction based on clinical assessment and its correlation with hospital mortality

		Case Fatality
Class 1	No failure	6%
Class 2	Mild – moderate heart failure (S3, crepitations	
	< 50% lung fields)	17%
Class 3	Severe heart failure (S3, crepitations > 50%	
	lung fields)	38%
Class 4	Cardiogenic shock	81%

3. An extensive MI has occurred
4. Abnormal chest x-ray (upper lobe diversion, Kerley B lines, cardiomegaly, alveolar oedema).

Although diagnosis and treatment are usually based on rapid clinical assessment, a more accurate evaluation of ventricular function can be obtained using echocardiography and pulmonary artery pressure monitoring. However, one should not delay immediate therapy, as these investigations may not always be appropriate and, if indicated, may be more helpful once the acute crisis has passed.

First line therapy

Most patients respond to first line treatment with diamorphine, loop diuretics (e.g. frusemide) and nitrates, as detailed below. Intravenous diamorphine is beneficial, both for its sedative effects and because it acts as a venodilator. Intravenous loop diuretics have a biphasic effect, with initial improvement in pre-load due to venodilatation followed by the onset of a diuresis. Reduction in cardiac pre-load and after-load with intravenous nitrates is beneficial where an adequate systolic blood pressure is present.

Initial treatment for LVF is as follows:

1. Sit the patient up.
2. Give high concentration oxygen therapy. If COPD is present, with its attendant risk of carbon dioxide retention, check blood gases and give controlled oxygen therapy starting at 24 or 28 per cent.
3. Give diamorphine 2.5 mg initially, by slow IV injection, and metoclopramide 10 mg and repeat the dose of diamorphine after five minutes if necessary.
4. Give IV frusemide 50–100 mg.

5. If systolic BP is above 100 mmHg, give 500 mcg of sublingual GTN and then commence an intravenous nitrate infusion as detailed in Chapter 24, increasing the infusion rate to the maximum haemodynamically tolerated dose if left ventricular failure is severe.

6. Correct any precipitating arrhythmias or ongoing ischaemia that may be present.

Patients require intensive monitoring, ideally in the Coronary Care Unit, which should include pulse oximetry (if available) and hourly urine output (via an indwelling urinary catheter). Routine bloods (including electrolytes, blood count, random glucose, cardiac enzymes), ECG and CXR should be performed in all cases.

Second line therapy

If initial treatment with diamorphine, frusemide and nitrates fails, then:

1. Give further diamorphine if the patient is still distressed.

2. Give further IV frusemide in double dose. **NB**: Frusemide will be ineffective if the renal blood flow is inadequate; thus there may not be a diuresis if the LVF is associated with hypotension, and additional drug therapy to raise blood pressure and improve renal blood flow may be necessary.

3. Consider inotropic support with dobutamine 5–20 mcg/kg/min and/or dopamine 2.5–5.0 mcg/kg/min if blood pressure drops below 100 mmHg or urine output falls below 30 ml/hour, for two consecutive hours.

4. Occasionally there may be marked bronchospasm (wheeze). This may be treated with bronchodilators such as salbutamol; however, this can be arrhythmogenic and the smallest effective dose should be used.

5. In patients who fail to respond to these measures, assisted ventilation may be helpful. This can be administered as:

   a. Continuous positive airways pressure (CPAP)
   b. Positive end expiratory pressure (PEEP)
   c. Intubation and assisted ventilation.

   Consult a senior colleague before instituting ventilation.

6. Look for treatable mechanical problems (Chapter 13). Severe mitral regurgitation or ventricular septal rupture should be excluded by an urgent bedside echocardiogram if suspected in patients with severe LVF.

Advice from a senior colleague should be sought if the patient has severe LVF due to a mechanical complication of myocardial infarction. In this situation, positive pressure ventilation or mechanical support (by the insertion of an intra-aortic balloon pump) may improve the patient's condition prior to cardiac catheterization with a view to early corrective surgery. Selective phosphodiesterase inhibitors, e.g. enoximone, which can be used in combination with dobutamine, may be beneficial in the short-term management of acute LVF. These work by increasing stroke volume and cardiac output by increasing inotropy while decreasing systemic and pulmonary vascular resistance, without altering heart rate. They may cause a substantial reduction in arterial pressure, and are contraindicated if the systolic pressure is below 90 mmHg. Invasive haemodynamic assessment (via a pulmonary artery pressure catheter) is required to monitor their use.

If the patient fails to respond to the above measures and there are no obvious reversible causes of LVF, the outlook is poor, as failure to respond frequently implies severe ventricular impairment.

Once patients have been stabilized they need to be switched to oral therapy for long-term control of heart failure. As a result of the AIRE study, patients with severe post-infarction heart failure have been shown to be the most likely to benefit from ACE inhibitor therapy (see Chapter 12). Although patients with severe LVF are more likely to suffer hypotension, particularly if they have received intensive diuretic therapy, treatment should be initiated as early as possible. In these cases it may be wise to start with a low dose short acting agent such as captopril, and titrate the dose upwards to the maximum tolerated dosage.

Key points

- The occurrence of LVF is most common after an anterior infarction, and is indicative of extensive myocardial damage.

- Patients who do not respond to first line therapy and who have no easily reversible cause of their heart failure have a poor prognosis.

- Positive pressure ventilation or mechanical support is worth considering where a reversible cause of the left ventricular failure exists and drug therapy has failed.

References

Diuretics for heart failure. (1994). *DTB*, **32,** 83–85.

Guidelines for the evaluation and management of heart failure. Report of the American College of Cardiology/American Heart Association Task Force on

Practice Guidelines (Committee on Evaluation and Management of Heart Failure). (1995). *J. Am. Coll. Cardiol.*, **26**, 1376–1398.

Johnston, S. and Watkins, J. (1988). Acute Heart Failure. *Hosp. Upd.*, 1578–1595.

Killip, T. and Kimball, J. T. (1967). Treatment of myocardial infarction in a coronary care unit; a two year experience with 250 patients. *Am. J. Cardiol.*, **20**, 457–464.

Raisanen, J., Heikkila, J., Downs, J., *et al.* (1985). Continuous positive airway pressure by face mask in acute cardiogenic pulmonary oedema. *Am. J. Cardiol.*, **55**, 296–300.

The AIRE study investigators. (1993). Effect of ramipril on mortality and morbidity of survivors of acute myocardial infarction with clinical evidence of heart failure. *Lancet*, **342**, 821–828.

Vismara, L. A., Ledman, D. M. and Zelis, R. (1976). The effects of morphine on venous tone in patients with acute pulmonary oedema. *Circulation*, **54**, 335–337.

Waller, D. (1994). Nitrates in the management of heart failure. *Br. J. Cardiol.*, 209–211.

11

Cardiogenic shock

Background

Cardiogenic shock is common following acute MI, occurring in 5–10 per cent of patients and accounting for the majority of in-hospital deaths. Cardiogenic shock is more common in older patients, diabetics (or patients with hyperglycaemia on admission), females and patients with a history of previous MI, and usually develops within 24 hours of admission. In 85 per cent of patients, cardiogenic shock is due to ischaemic damage to more than 40 per cent of the left ventricle associated with extensive anterior infarction, or a more limited infarction in a patient with pre-existing ischaemic ventricular dysfunction. In some patients, a vicious cycle of initial hypotension produces reduced coronary perfusion, further ischaemia and necrosis leading to infarct extension and progressive left ventricular dysfunction. In 15 per cent of patients cardiogenic shock is due to potentially reversible complications such as right ventricular infarction, ventricular septal defect or severe mitral regurgitation; these patients tend to develop cardiogenic shock after the first 24 hours, and need to be accurately identified to facilitate appropriate treatment.

The prognosis of cardiogenic shock treated with conventional medical therapy is poor, with an in-hospital mortality rate of 80 per cent or more. Thrombolytic therapy usually fails to achieve reperfusion of the infarct-related artery in patients who develop cardiogenic shock, and has had no significant effect on prognosis. Supportive therapy with ionotropic agents may produce a temporary improvement in the haemodynamic state, but has no beneficial effect on survival.

Recent evidence from studies containing around 4000 patients in total (including 3000 patients with cardiogenic shock prospectively studied in the GUSTO-1 study) suggests that early (within 24 hours) aggressive supportive therapy utilizing intra-aortic balloon pumps (IABPs), right heart catheterization, ventilatory support and cardiac catheterization with PTCA in patients with suitable anatomy will improve the likelihood of survival. Restoration of adequate flow to the infarct territory by PTCA (with stenting if necessary) may be the most effective treatment for cardiogenic shock. The pooled data suggests that successful PTCA with restoration of adequate flow in the infarct-related artery can be achieved in 75 per cent of patients catheterized for cardiogenic shock. Failure to achieve patency of the infarct-related artery is associated with a poor prognosis. Patients in whom PTCA is successful have an in-hospital mortality rate of 25–30 per cent, with more than 50 per cent of patients surviving for one year with an acceptable quality of life. Although this data needs to be confirmed in a randomized trial, it does suggest that, if local facilities and expertise permit, PTCA should be considered for appropriate patients who develop cardiogenic shock following acute MI. As yet, there is no data that will allow us to identify those patients who will gain most from aggressive treatment to improve haemodynamics and restore adequate flow in the infarct-related artery.

Diagnosis of cardiogenic shock

Features associated with cardiogenic shock due to severe left ventricular dysfunction include:

1. Persistent hypotension (systolic BP < 90 mmHg)

2. Clinical signs of a low output state (urine output < 30 ml/hour, poor peripheral perfusion, or impaired cerebration)

3. Evidence of raised cardiac filling pressures (the presence of clinical or radiological evidence of pulmonary oedema implies that the pulmonary artery wedge pressure is > 15 mmHg).

It is important to exclude other causes of hypotension and potentially reversible complications of acute MI. If the patient has:

1. A late onset of cardiogenic shock (more than 24 hours after admission), or develops a new murmur, when the haemodynamic impairment may be secondary to a ventricular septal defect or severe mitral regurgitation

2. Hypotension in the absence of clinical or radiological evidence of pulmonary oedema, particularly if associated with inferior or posterior infarction, when the haemodynamic impairment may be secondary to right ventricular infarction

3. Hypotension in association with a poor fluid intake or aggressive diuretic

therapy, when the haemodynamic impairment may be secondary to intravascular volume depletion.

A senior colleague should be contacted, as insertion of a pulmonary artery catheter and urgent echocardiography may be necessary to rule out treatable problems.

Management of cardiogenic shock due to severe left ventricular dysfunction

The management of cardiogenic shock due to severe left ventricular impairment is as follows:

1. Treat arrhythmias, correct hypoxia with oxygen, control pain with diamorphine and correct hyperglycaemia with insulin. Treat pulmonary oedema with intravenous frusemide.

2. Attempt to stabilize or improve the haemodynamic state with inotropes. Give dobutamine 5–20 mcg/kg/min intravenously (via a peripheral line) to increase cardiac output and dopamine 2.5–5.0 mcg/kg/min (via a central line) to improve renal blood flow (see Chapter 24 for infusion details). If no haemodynamic improvement occurs, consider a noradrenaline infusion in selected patients.

3. Discuss urgent cardiac catheterization with a senior colleague, with a view to PTCA in appropriate patients. Insertion of an IABP prior to PTCA may help to improve cardiac output and coronary diastolic flow, decreasing the rate of early infarct-related artery re-occlusion and recurrent ischaemia. A pulmonary artery catheter will help to optimize cardiac function, and ventilation may improve gas exchange prior to PTCA.

It is also important to clearly explain to patients' relatives the poor prognosis associated with cardiogenic shock.

Management of cardiogenic shock due to right ventricular infarction

Significant hypotension can occur in association with right ventricular dysfunction due to extensive inferoposterior infarction. Unlike cardiogenic shock due to extensive left ventricular dysfunction, prognosis with appropriate treatment is relatively good, with mortality rates of around 20 per cent.

Right ventricular infarction should be suspected when hypotension occurs in a patient with clear lung fields and a raised JVP. If right ventricular infarction is suspected, record a V4R lead. The presence of 1 mm ST elevation in this lead is diagnostic of right ventricular infarction, but this is often a transient finding and its absence does not exclude the diagnosis. If any diagnostic doubt exists, consult a senior colleague. Insertion of a pulmonary artery catheter will help to clarify the situation if necessary. The characteristic haemodynamic pattern shows a low or normal wedge pressure, with an elevated right ventricular diastolic and right atrial pressure. Treatment consists of administering intravenous fluids rapidly (200 ml of normal saline over 10 minutes followed by 1–2 l over four hours, followed by an infusion of 1 l every six hours may be needed, with the fluid regime adjusted to maintain wedge pressure at 15 mmHg) to increase the right ventricular pre-load and thereby raise cardiac output. Diuretics and vasodilators will have an adverse effect on haemodynamic function and should be avoided. If hypotension persists after appropriate fluid loading, treat with dobutamine 5–20 mcg/kg/min. Right ventricular infarction is complicated by arrhythmias in 30–50 per cent of patients. If AF occurs, this should be corrected promptly, as the atrial contribution to right ventricular filling is important in this context. If heart block develops, dual chamber pacing is necessary to maintain atrioventricular synchrony.

Management of cardiogenic shock due to mechanical complications

Patients with a VSD or severe mitral regurgitation complicating an acute MI often develop cardiogenic shock. These complications should be excluded in all patients, particularly if new murmurs are present or cardiogenic shock develops after the first 24 hours, and echocardiography is mandatory in these circumstances. The management of these patients is discussed in more detail in Chapter 13.

Management of hypotension due to intravascular volume depletion

In some patients who have been treated with aggressive diuretic therapy, or in whom fluid intake is less than output, intravascular volume depletion may lead to post-infarction hypotension. These patients will have a low blood pressure in the absence of signs of pulmonary oedema or right ventricular infarction. If any doubt exists, insertion of a pulmonary artery catheter will clarify the underlying diagnosis; wedge pressure, right ventricular and atrial pressures will all be low. Volume replacement rather than ionotropic therapy is the treatment of choice.

Key points

- Cardiogenic shock is a common and often lethal complication of acute MI.

- Supportive therapy with ionotropes has no effect on the high mortality rate.

- PTCA and intensive supportive therapy with pulmonary artery catheters, IABP and ventilation if necessary improves outcome, and should be considered in selected cases.

- Patients who develop haemodynamic problems after the first 24 hours, particularly if they occur in association with inferior infarction or new murmurs, or in the absence of pulmonary oedema, may have a mechanical complication, right ventricular infarction or relative hypovolaemia. Insertion of a pulmonary artery catheter will clarify the diagnosis and help to guide treatment in these patients.

References

Barnard, M. J., Linter, S.P.K. (1993). Acute circulatory support. *Br. Med. J.*, **307**, 35–41.

Califf, R. M. and Bengtson, J. R. (1994). Cardiogenic shock. *N. Engl. J. Med.*, **330**, 1724–1730.

Eltehaninaff, H., Simpfendorfer, C., Franco, I., *et al.* (1995). Early and one year survival rates in acute MI complicated by cardiogenic shock: A retrospective study comparing coronary angioplasty with medical treatment. *Am. Heart J.*, **130**, 459–464.

Hochman, J. S., Boland, J., Sleeper, J. A., *et al.* (1995). Current spectrum of cardiogenic shock and effect of early revascularization on mortality. *Circulation*, **91**, 873–881.

Holmes, D. R., Butes, E. R., Kleiman, N. S. *et al.* (1995). Contemporary reperfusion therapy for cardiogenic shock: the GUSTO-1 trial experience. *J. Am. Coll. Cardiol.*, **26**, 668–674.

Holmes, D. R. and Topel, E. J. (1997). Cardiogenic shock: 'going to the mat' – is it needed and does it work? *Eur. Heart J.*, **18**, 1839–1840.

Holmes, D. R., Califf, R. M., Vau de Werf, F. *et al.* (1997). Differences in countries' use of resources and clinical outcome for patients with cardiogenic shock after MI: results from the GUSTO trial. *Lancet*, **349**, 75–78.

Kinch, J. W. and Ryan, T. J. (1994). Right ventricular infarction. *N. Engl. J. Med.*, **330**, 1211–1217.

Richard, C., Ricome, J. C., Rimailho, A. *et al.* (1982). Combined haemodynamic effects of dopamine and dobutamine in cardiogenic shock. *Circulation*, **67**, 620–626.

12

ACE inhibitors following acute myocardial infarction

Background

Angiotensin converting enzyme (ACE) inhibitors were initially introduced for the treatment of hypertension. They have subsequently become established in the treatment of heart failure and, more recently, for post-MI patients. This latter indication arose from animal and human studies which demonstrated that ACE inhibitors have beneficial effects on left ventricular remodelling after MI.

The process of remodelling starts in the early hours following an infarction. Infarct expansion occurs as the affected heart muscle stretches and thins, which may result in cardiac rupture or aneurysm formation. To compensate for the area of impaired function, the remaining viable myocardium undergoes hypertrophy and the chamber size increases. This global ventricular dilatation is a powerful predictor of mortality.

ACE inhibitors work by blocking the conversion of angiotensin I to angiotensin II, the actions of which are numerous and diverse. In particular, angiotensin II is a potent vasoconstrictor (which will increase afterload), it can act as a growth factor (resulting in hypertrophy), it may be toxic to myocytes, it modulates sympathetic nerve activity and increases aldosterone production (increasing sodium and water retention). These are some of the mechanisms by which ACE inhibitors are thought to exert their influence and be of benefit following MI.

In clinical trials, approximately 100 000 patients have been randomized to receive an ACE inhibitor post-MI. A summary of the major trials is presented in Table 12.1, followed by a brief synopsis of their results.

In CONSENSUS II, all patients with MI in the absence of hypotension were eligible to be randomized to IV ACE inhibition (enalaprilat), followed by long-term oral therapy. This study of early, unselected ACE inhibition was abandoned, as the data showed no significant

Table 12.1 ACE inhibitor trials post MI. (EF = ejection fraction.)

Study	Number	Entry criteria post-MI
CONSENSUS II	6090	all patients, <24 hours
SAVE	2231	EF <40%, 3–16 days
AIRE	2006	clinical heart failure, 3–10 days
GISSI-3	18 895	all patients, <24 hours
ISIS-4	58 043	all patients, <24 hours
SMILE	1556	non-thrombolized anterior MIs, <24 hours
TRACE	1749	LV dysfunction, 3–7 days
Chinese Cardiac Study	13 634	all patients, <36 hours

reduction in mortality in the ACE inhibitor group at six months. In the SAVE study, asymptomatic patients were randomized to captopril at a mean of 11 days post-MI if they had an ejection fraction of <40 per cent, as assessed by radionuclide ventriculography. This was the first study to show a conclusive reduction in mortality (19 per cent) with the use of an ACE inhibitor post-MI, although the effect was only seen after a minimum two year follow up. The AIRE Study investigated the use of ACE inhibitors (ramipril) in the 15 per cent to 20 per cent of patients who develop clinically evident heart failure following infarction. Treatment was commenced a mean five days post-MI in this selected population. The risk reduction in mortality was substantial at 27 per cent after an average 15 months of treatment, and the benefit appeared rapidly, approaching significance at only 30 days after randomization.

The results of these earlier studies were examined in the large mega-trials of ISIS-4, GISSI-3 and the Chinese Cardiac Study, which together randomized over 89 000 patients to early (within 36 hours) ACE inhibitor treatment or control. All patients with MI in the absence of hypotension were eligible. Early, non-selective, oral ACE inhibition produced a small (seven per cent) risk reduction in mortality at four to six weeks. Sub-group analysis suggested that most of this mortality reduction was due to the treatment of high risk patients, such as those with extensive infarction or clinically evident heart failure. There was very little mortality reduction in low risk groups.

More recently, the SMILE study examined the role of early ACE inhibition (zofenopril) in patients with anterior MI not suitable for thrombolysis. Follow up at one year, despite cessation of therapy after only six weeks, showed a mortality benefit of 29 per cent. The TRACE study showed that in selected patients with echocardiographic evidence of left ventricular dysfunction, there was a risk reduction in mortality of 22 per cent with long-term treatment (two to four years). Again, like the AIRE study, benefit was shown even by one month of treatment. The most recently published mortality data with ACE inhibitors post-MI came from the AIRE Extension (AIREX) study. All patients recruited from the UK for the original AIRE study were followed up for a mean period of almost five years. Those treated with ramipril compared to placebo had a relative risk reduction in mortality of 36 per cent during long-term follow up.

The benefits from ACE inhibitor treatment are now clearly established in patients with left ventricular dysfunction or heart failure post-MI. These studies indicate that:

1. Patients with clinically evident heart failure post-MI have a large mortality reduction with ACE inhibitor therapy (AIRE study), which is sustained over many years (AIREX study).

2. Patients with significant left ventricular dysfunction post-MI (assessed by echo or isotope ventriculography) have a large mortality reduction with ACE inhibitor therapy (SAVE, TRACE studies).

3. Very early (within 24 hours) IV ACE inhibition is of no benefit (CONSENSUS II).

4. Early (within 36 hours) non-selective ACE inhibition of all post-infarct patients is safe if patients with hypotension are excluded, but is associated with only a small mortality reduction (ISIS-4, GISSI-3 and Chinese Cardiac Study). This is likely to be due to the treatment of high risk patients with extensive infarction and heart failure; low risk patients probably benefit little from ACE inhibitor therapy.

5. Patients with asymptomatic left ventricular dysfunction can be identified by echocardiography during their convalescent phase, and show a large mortality reduction if treated with ACE inhibitors (TRACE).

Inclusion criteria

On the basis of these results, we recommend that all post-infarct patients should at least be considered for ACE inhibitor therapy. Treatment should then be targeted to those with clinical heart failure, significant left ventricular impairment or extensive infarction, so as to reduce mortality in high risk groups. Low risk patients (those with small infarcts, no clinical evidence of heart failure and well preserved left ventricular function) stand to gain little from ACE inhibitor therapy. If in doubt, assess left ventricular function by echocardiography. Patients with an ejection fraction of less than 40 per cent should be treated. ACE inhibitors can be combined with beta-blockade to provide additional benefit through complementary mechanisms. However, tolerance of this regime will depend on the degree of left ventricular dysfunction and the presence of on-going ischaemia or arrhythmias, and will require careful monitoring.

We recommend that treatment is commenced once the patient is clinically stable, usually within 48 hours of infarction. Treatment may be started with a low dose of a long acting agent (e.g. ramipril 2.5 mg daily or lisinopril 2.5 mg daily) increasing to the recommended dose (ramipril 10 mg daily or lisinopril 10 mg daily) over two to four days. This dosage titration is of particular importance, as lower doses of ACE inhibitors have not been evaluated in clinical trials, and may not provide the same level of mortality and morbidity benefit.

If the patient is at high risk of first dose hypotension (systolic BP less than 100 mmHg, on large doses of diuretics, or hypovolaemic), a low dose of a short acting agent (captopril 6.25 mg) can be used. Maximum blood pressure fall should be within one hour. The choice of subsequent dose or change to a low dose of long acting agent depends on response. Patients who are susceptible to hypotension should have their diuretics omitted for 24 hours before commencement of ACE inhibition, and the first dose administered in the evening.

Exclusion criteria

1. Supine BP less than 90 mmHg systolic
2. Significant valve stenosis
3. History of angio-oedema or sensitivity to ACE inhibitors
4. Severe renal, hepatic or haematological disorders (especially renal artery stenosis)
5. History of cerebral ischaemia related to hypotension
6. Pregnancy or porphyria.

Administration regime

1. Give ramipril 2.5 mg or equivalent, and monitor BP at one hourly intervals.
2. If systolic BP remains above 90 mmHg after 12 hours, commence ramipril 5 mg daily (or equivalent), increasing to a maintenance dose of 10 mg daily if possible.

3. The initial dose can be reduced to 1.25 mg if there are concerns about hypotension.

NB: Electrolytes should be checked before starting therapy and monitored during treatment to ensure that renal impairment is not developing. Concomitant treatment with non-steroidal anti-inflammatory agents increases the risk of renal damage. Potassium-sparing diuretics should generally be changed to a non-potassium sparing equivalent. Treatment should be continued long-term unless a side-effect develops or the patient's clinical condition changes.

Recent data from the ELITE study suggests that AII receptor blockers may be useful in patients who are intolerant of ACE inhibitors. In this study, over 700 patients were randomized to captopril or the AII receptor blocker losartan. Losartan was very well tolerated, with no withdrawals due to cough, rash, taste disturbance or angio-oedema. Death and hospitalization were less common in patients treated with losartan. Although these provisional results need to be confirmed in the larger scale and ongoing ELITE II study, they do suggest that when it is necessary to withdraw an ACE inhibitor, an AII receptor antagonist is a safe and effective alternative.

Key points

- ACE inhibitors should be given to all post-infarct patients with clinical evidence of heart failure and those with significant left ventricular impairment, even if asymptomatic.

- Patients with small infarcts and well preserved left ventricular function are at low risk of early mortality and probably do not derive great benefit from ACE inhibition.

- It is reasonable to introduce treatment once the patient is clinically stable (usually within 48 hours post-infarction), beginning with a low dose of a suitable agent and aiming to discharge the patient on a maintenance dose equivalent to that used in clinical trials.

References

Ambrostom, E. and Borghi, C. (1995). Magnam B for the survival of MI long-term evaluation, SMILE: study investigators. The effect of angiotensin converting enzyme inhibitor zofenopril on mortality and morbidity after anterior MI. *N. Engl. J. Med.*, **332**, 80–85.

GISSI-3 (Gruppo Italiano per lo Studio della Supravvivenza nell'Infarto Miocardico). (1994). Effects of lisinopril and transdermal glyceryl trinitrate singly and together on six-week mortality and ventricular function after acute MI. *Lancet*, **343**, 1115–1122.

Hall, A. S., Murray, G. D. and Ball, S. G. (1997). Follow up study of patients randomly allocated ramipril or placebo for heart failure after acute MI: AIRE Extension (AIREX) Study. *Lancet*, **349**, 1493–1497.

Hansson, L. (1997). ACE inhibition and left ventricular remodelling. *Eur. Heart J.*, **18**, 1203–1204.

ISIS-4 Collaborative Group. (1995). Fourth International Study of Infarct Survival. A randomized factorial trial assessing early oral captopril, oral mononitrate, and intravenous magnesium sulphate in 58 050 patients with suspected acute MI. *Lancet*, **345**, 669–685.

Kober, L., Torp-Pedersen, C., Carlsen, J. E., *et al.* (for the Trandolapril Cardiac Evaluation (TRACE) Study Group). (1995). A clinical trial of the angiotensin-converting enzyme inhibitor trandolapril in patients with left ventricular dysfunction after MI. *N. Engl. J. Med.*, **333**, 1670–1676.

Lisheng, L., Liu, L. S., Wang, W., *et al.* (for the Chinese Cardiac Study Collaborative Group). (1995). Oral captopril versus placebo among 13 634 patients with suspected acute MI: interim report from the Chinese Cardiac Study (CCS-1). *Lancet*, **345**, 680–687.

Pitts, B., Segal, R., Murtinez, F. A., *et al.* (1997). Randomized trial of losartan versus captopril in patients over 65 with heart failure (Evaluation of Losartan in the Elderly Study, ELITE). *Lancet*, **349**, 747–752.

Ptelter, M. A., Braunwald, E., Moye, L. A., *et al.* (on behalf of the SAVE Investigators). (1992). Effect of captopril on mortality and morbidity in patients with left ventricular dysfunction after MI. *N. Engl. J. Med.*, **327**, 669–677.

Swedberg, K., Held, P., Kjekshus, J., *et al.* (on behalf of the CONSENSUS II Study Group). (1992). Effects of the early administration of enalapril on mortality in patients with acute MI: Results of the Cooperative New Scandinavian Enalapril Survival Study II (CONSENSUS II). *N. Engl. J. Med.*, **327**, 678–684.

The Acute Infarction Ramipril Efficacy (AIRE) Study Investigators. (1993). Effect of ramipril on mortality and morbidity of survivors of acute MI with clinical evidence of heart failure. *Lancet*, **342**, 821–828.

13

Mechanical complications of acute myocardial infarction

Background

The commonest early complications of acute MI are heart failure and arrhythmias, dealt with in detail in Chapters 8, 10 and 11. The complications of cardiac rupture and severe mitral regurgitation are less common, but are associated with a high mortality. This mortality may be reduced if an appropriate referral for possible corrective surgery is made before established cardiogenic shock develops, and this chapter deals with the early diagnosis and management of these complications.

Rupture of the left ventricular free wall

Left ventricular free wall rupture occurs in around five per cent of all acute infarct patients, usually within the first week, and is the cause of death in around 20 per cent of patients with acute MI. It is more common in elderly female patients with a first anterolateral infarct and a history of hypertension. The incidence of free wall rupture may be increased by thrombolytic therapy, particularly if it is given late in the course of the infarct. Concomitant therapy with intravenous beta-blockers may reduce the risk of this complication. Most patients present with acute rupture, leading to cardiovascular collapse and electromechanical dissociation. Acute rupture of the left ventricular free wall is usually fatal, and does not respond to standard cardiopulmonary resuscitation. In 25 per cent of patients there may be a sub-acute presentation, with a slow leak or pericardial adhesions limiting the initial flow of blood into the pericardial space. These patients develop a cardiogenic shock picture with evidence of cardiac tamponade. The presence of pericardial fluid can rapidly be confirmed by bedside echocardiography. Aspiration of pericardial fluid may stabilize the haemodynamic state and allow the rupture to heal in some patients. Immediate surgery should be considered, irrespective of the clinical status of the patient, as an acute episode with electro-mechanical dissociation and death may follow.

Ventricular septal rupture

Rupture of the intraventricular septum occurs in one to two per cent of post-infarct patients, usually within the first week and in association with a transmural infarction, and it is a common cause of death in patients who suffer from MI. With anterior infarction, occlusion of the left anterior descending coronary artery usually produces a defect in the anterior or apical septum. Two-thirds of post-infarct septal ruptures are associated with anterior infarction. With inferior infarction, the defect is often sited in the inferior septum close to the mitral annulus. Patients with ventricular septal rupture present with cardiogenic shock in associa-tion with a new systolic murmur, loudest at the lower left sternal edge. The diagnosis can be confirmed by echocardiography and right heart catheterization. Without corrective surgery, 90 per cent of patients die within two weeks. When the diagnosis is confirmed, initial treatment is with inotropes and an IABP to try and achieve haemodynamic stability. Urgent coronary angiography is usually necessary, since almost 50 per cent of patients have associated multivessel coronary disease, and the outcome of surgery may be improved by additional coronary grafting (if possible, at the time of surgery). Surgical mortality is 25–50 per cent, and is highest in patients who are older (>70 years) or have established shock or renal impairment, and those with defects due to inferior infarcts (which are technically difficult to repair). It is therefore essential to contact a senior colleague as soon as you suspect a possible septal rupture, as early investigation and surgical referral offer the best hope of survival. Surgery should probably be carried out soon after the diagnosis is established, as delay usually leads to haemodynamic deterioration with multi-organ failure and decreases the chance of surviving an operation.

Mitral regurgitation

Acute MI is often associated with a minor degree of mitral regurgitation, which is tolerated with no significant haemodynamic impairment. The regurgitation is often associated with left ventricular dilatation and is reversible with appropriate therapy. Severe mitral regurgitation due to papillary muscle rupture complicates around one per cent of infarcts, usually during the first post-infarct week. Most patients with papillary muscle rupture have breathlessness and haemodynamic compromise associated with a new apical systolic murmur. The haemodynamic state may be stabilized by inotropes and an IABP, but mortality is 50 per cent within 24 hours and 94 per cent by eight weeks without surgical intervention. The diagnosis is confirmed by a combination of echocardiography and right heart catheterization. Early surgical intervention reduces mortality to around 30 per cent.

Investigation of patients with possible ventricular septal rupture or severe mitral regurgitation

All patients who develop unexpected haemodynamic problems in association with a new systolic murmur following MI should be immediately discussed with a senior colleague. Although inotropes, diuretics and IABP may stabilize the haemodynamic state in the short-term, progressive heart failure and death usually occur without corrective surgery. A delay in establishing the diagnosis may compromise surgical outcome, which is much worse in patients with established cardiogenic shock or renal impairment. A combination of clinical assessment, echocardiography and right heart catheterization with oximetry will usually establish the diagnosis (Table 13.1). Coronary angiography may be necessary after discussing the case with cardiac surgeons, if it is felt that additional coronary bypass surgery will be feasible or advantageous.

Table 13.1 Differentiation of ventricular septal rupture from acute severe mitral regurgitation.

	Ventricular septal rupture	Acute severe mitral regurgitation
Murmur	Usually loudest at lower left sternal edge	Usually loudest at apex, radiates to axilla
Site of infarct	Anterior or inferior	Usually inferior
2-D echo-cardiography	Defect in intraventricular septum may be visible	Ruptured papillary muscles or a flail mitral leaflet may be visible
Doppler echo-cardiography	A turbulent jet crossing the intraventricular septum from left to right ventricle may be visible. A high velocity jet implies a small defect, a low velocity jet a large defect	Prominent regurgitant flow from left ventricle to left atrium visible. An increase in mitral forward flow to $>2\,\text{m/s}$ or systolic flow reversal

		in the pulmonary veins implies severe regurgitation
Right heart catheterization and oximetry	An increase in oxygen saturation of >10% in the right ventricle compared to right atrium, due to oxygenated blood crossing the septal defect. A large increase in saturation implies a large defect	No step up in oxygen saturation. Prominent V-waves may be visible in the pulmonary artery wedge trace in severe mitral regurgitation

Key points

- Rupture of the left ventricular free wall is an important cause of sudden death early after acute MI.

- Sub-acute rupture presenting with tamponade requires consideration of immediate surgery.

- Ventricular septal defect is an important cause of post-infarction in-hospital death. Surgery carries a high mortality (particularly in the elderly, if the VSD occurs in association with an inferior infarct, or if cardiogenic shock or renal impairment is present preoperatively), but offers the only hope of survival.

- Acute severe mitral regurgitation can usually be diagnosed on the basis of echocardiography and right heart catheterization. Early surgery offers the best hope of survival.

References

Bates, R. J., Beutler, S., Resnekov, L., *et al.* (1997). Cardiac rupture: challenge in management. *Am. J. Cardiol.*, **42**, 429–437.

Cohn, O. H. (1991). Surgical management of acute and chronic cardiac and mechanical complications due to MI. *Am. Heart J.*, **102**, 1049–1060.

Nishimura, R. A., Schaff, H. V., Shub, C., *et al.* (1983). Papillary muscle rupture complicating acute MI. *Am. J. Cardiol.*, **51**, 373–377.

O'Rourke, M. (1973). Sub-acute heart rupture following acute MI. *Lancet*, **2**, 124–126.

Pellerin, M. and Bourassa, M. G. (1996). Post-infarction ventricular septal rupture. *Eur. Heart J.*, **17**, 1778–1779.

Radford, M. J., Johnson, R. A., Duggett, W. M. J. *et al.* (1991). Ventricular septal rupture: a review of clinical physiological features and an analysis of survival. *Circulation*, **64**, 545–553.

Stryjer, D., Friedensohn, A. and Hendler, A. (1988). Myocardial rupture in acute myocardial infarction: urgent management. *Br. Heart J.*, **59**, 73–74.

Sutherland, F. W. H., Guell, F. J., Pathi, V., *et al.* (1996). Post-infarction ventricular free wall rupture; strategies for diagnosis and treatment. *Ann. Thorac. Surg.*, **61**, 1281–1285.

14

The in-hospital convalescent phase of acute myocardial infarction

Background

Following admission with acute MI, most patients should remain on bed rest for 12–24 hours. In uncomplicated cases, the patient can sit out of bed and undertake self-care within 24 hours. Patients who have a relatively limited infarct with no sustained high grade arrhythmias, heart failure or continuing ischaemia are at low risk of in-hospital complications, and should be transferred out of the CCU environment after 24 hours. Patients who have complications should be kept on bed rest in the CCU until their clinical condition stabilizes. Patients with an uncomplicated course can be discharged within one week; those with complications will need a longer period of hospitalization. In addition to the major life-threatening in-hospital complications of arrhythmias, cardiogenic shock, cardiac rupture and mitral regurgitation, a variety of other problems can arise during the convalescent phase of acute MI, and these are dealt with in this chapter.

Thromboembolic complications

Clinically significant deep venous thrombosis and pulmonary embolism (PE) are now rare following MI. Patients who have complicated infarcts with a prolonged period of bed rest are most at risk. Prophylactic low dose subcutaneous heparin (5000 units bd) should be instituted in high risk patients, to minimize the occurrence of venous thromboembolism. Intraventricular thrombus formation may occur following acute infarction, and is associated with an increased risk of thromboembolism. Inferior infarction is associated with a low risk, but 30–40 per cent of patients with anterior infarction will have echocardiographically detectable left ventricular thrombus, and are at increased risk of embolic stroke. The risk of stroke can be substantially reduced by anticoagulants, and is maximal in the first three months after infarction. All patients with extensive anterior infarction should be screened by echocardiography. In the absence of contraindications, the finding of a protuberant mobile thrombus or significant left ventricular dysfunction is an indication to consider warfarin therapy, which should be continued long term.

Post-infarction pericarditis

Pericarditis can complicate infarction in any site. In pericarditis complicating anterior infarction, the pain is usually typical, well localized and often associated with a friction rub. In inferior infarction, the pain may be atypical in site and is not usually associated with a rub, and may therefore present diagnostic difficulties. Patients who develop pericarditis usually have extensive infarction and an adverse prognosis. Progression of pericarditis to a clinically significant effusion is rare. Treatment should be with simple analgesic agents such as paracetamol or dihydrocodeine, with non-steroidal anti-inflammatory agents reserved for patients with severe or persistent pericarditis. Dressler's syndrome tends to occur much later, and is now rare. Patients present with pain, a pericardial friction rub, raised inflammatory markers, fever and pleurisy. Most patients with Dressler's syndrome will require treatment with a short course of steroids.

Recurrent ischaemia

The occurrence of persistent or recurrent ischaemic chest pain with electrocardiographic changes is often associated with progressive ventricular damage, re-occlusion of the infarct-related artery and a high risk of early morbidity and mortality. When recurrent ischaemia occurs treatment is as follows:

1. Relieve pain and anxiety with intravenous diamorphine

2. If ST elevation occurs in association with recurrent symptoms, contact a senior colleague to discuss treatment options aimed at restoring patency in the infarct-related artery (options are further thrombolysis or urgent PTCA)

3. If ST depression occurs, commence on nitrate and heparin infusions and contact a senior colleague to arrange early angiography with a view to assessing revascularization options.

Depending on the results of angiography, PTCA or CABG may be necessary to stabilize the patient's condition.

Left ventricular aneurysm

Infarct expansion leading to aneurysm formation usually occurs in association with a persistently occluded left anterior descending coronary artery in a patient who presents with extensive anterior infarction. The electrocardiogram often shows persistent ST elevation. These patients often have a complicated in-hospital course with an increased risk of heart failure, late arrhythmias and thromboembolism. Careful screening to establish the need for revascularization, anticoagulation and therapy designed to limit the risk of arrhythmic death is indicated, as discussed in detail in Chapter 15.

Late ventricular arrythmias

Ventricular arrhythmias that occur after the first 24 hours are associated with large infarctions, and are liable to recur. As discussed in Chapters 8 and 15, these patients require careful evaluation by an electrophysiologist to determine the most appropriate treatment strategy.

Key points

- Early mobilization and discharge within a week is appropriate for patients with uncomplicated infarction.

- Thromboembolic complications are more common in patients with large infarctions. Patients with extensive anterior infarctions should be screened for intraventricular thrombus to determine the need for warfarin.

- Clinically evident pericarditis is usually associated with large anterior infarcts. Pericarditis complicating inferior infarction may be atypical, and is more difficult to diagnose.

- Recurrent ischaemia in the early post-infarction phase usually requires the re-establishment of intravenous anti-ischaemic therapy and urgent angiography to assess the indications for revascularization.

References

Goldstein, S. (1993). Early discharge after a MI: what's the hurry? *J. Am. Coll. Cardiol.*, **22**, 1802–1803.

Loh, E. and St John Sutton, M. (1997). Anticoagulation and left ventricular dysfunction: friend or foe? *Eur. Heart J.*, **18**, 1039–1041.

McNeer, J., Wagner, G., Ginsburg, P., *et al.* (1978). Hospital discharge one week after acute MI. *N. Engl. J. Med.*, **2948**, 229–232.

Thompson, P. L. and Robinson, J. S. (1978). Stroke after acute MI: relation to infarct size. *Br. Med. J.*, **1**, 457–459.

Tofler, G. H., Muller, J. E., Stone, P. H., *et al.* (1989). Pericarditis in acute MI: characterization and clinical significance. *Am. Heart J.*, **117**, 86–92.

Visser, C. A., Kan, G., Meltzer, R. S., *et al.* (1985). Embolic potential of left ventricular thrombus after MI: a two dimensional echocardiographic study of 119 patients. *J. Am. Coll. Cardiol.*, **5**, 1276–1280.

15

Risk stratification and management during the recovery phase of acute myocardial infarction

Background

In the last 30 years, modern therapy for acute MI has halved in-hospital mortality in younger patients. However, patients who survive their infarct are at increased risk of cardiac events in subsequent years. Risk stratification and secondary prevention measures are important to improve prognosis, and the remainder of this chapter will give guidelines on treatment and investigation of infarct survivors.

Lifestyle and rehabilitation

At least a quarter of infarct survivors suffer clinically important psycho-logical problems. Early advice and literature on lifestyle modification and self-help are effective in reducing early distress in the majority of patients. Those with more severe emotional reactions to an infarction should be referred for formal psychiatric assessment. If available locally, referral to a cardiac rehabilitation program is of value in improving quality of life, and may improve long-term survival. Patients should optimally be reviewed by a dietician, and a reducing diet should be prescribed for those who are overweight. Switching to a diet low in fat and high in fibre, oily fish, fruit and vegetables may also help to reduce mortality. Consumption of small amounts of alcohol (less than three units a day) may have some cardioprotective effect, but a high intake of alcohol is associated with hypertension and increased mortality, and should be discouraged. Stopping smoking is an effective way to reduce the risk of further cardiac events. Mortality in infarct survivors who give up smoking is reduced by 50 per cent, and the prevalence of post-infarction angina is also reduced. Nicotine replacement therapy helps in smoking cessation, and can be safely used in the presence of coronary artery disease. Information and support for smokers trying to give up can be obtained from Action on Smoking and Health (0171 935 3519), Quit (0171 487 2858), the Health Education Authority (0171 383 3833) and the British Medical Association (0171 383 6625). The risk of recurrent cardiac events remains high in patients who cannot stop smoking and can only reduce the number of cigarettes smoked, or switch to low tar cigarettes, cigars or a pipe. Passive smoking increases the risk of ischaemic heart disease by around 30 per cent, and partners of infarct survivors should be encouraged to stop. The risk of smoking one cigarette per day or of chronic exposure to passive smoking is equivalent to half the risk associated with smoking 20 cigarettes per day.

Following discharge from hospital, patients should be encouraged to gradually increase their level of physical activity over four to six weeks. If a post-infarct exercise test is satisfactory, patients can then resume normal activity, including returning to work if appropriate. Patients should be instructed to inform their motor vehicle insurance companies after recent MIs. Driving can be resumed four weeks after an uncomplicated infarct without informing the DVLA. If the patient has heart failure, dangerous arrhythmias or angina precipitated by driving, advice on resuming driving must be taken from the DVLA. Licences for driving heavy goods vehicles and public service vehicles are automatically withdrawn, and the patient must inform the DVLA of a recent infarction. In some circumstances an HGV licence may be regained, and it is the patient's responsibility to negotiate this with the DVLA, who will request relevant information from the hospital. Sexual activity should be avoided for two to three weeks. Patients with a satisfactory exercise test can be reassured that cardiovascular demands during intercourse are normally less than those during an exercise test. Air travel should be avoided for six weeks after an uncomplicated infarct, or longer in patients with heart failure or severe angina.

Pharmacological secondary prevention

Most patients will be commenced on aspirin and a beta-blocker in the first 48 hours after admission with acute MI. In the absence of side-effects, beta-blockers should be continued indefinitely, as withdrawal may precipitate episodes of rebound ischaemia. If a beta-blocker is contra-indicated, a calcium antagonist such as verapamil or diltiazem is an alternative in patients with well preserved left ventricular function. Patients who have had clinical evidence of heart failure or evidence of an extensive infarct will normally receive an ACE inhibitor prior to discharge from CCU. In these patients, the dose of ACE inhibitor should be titrated upwards to the levels used in post-infarction mortality trials (10 mg daily of ramipril, 10 mg of lisinopril and 50–100 mg daily of captopril) if these doses are tolerated, and continued indefinitely. Patients who have no clinical evidence of heart failure should have an echocardiogram, and those who have evidence of significant asymptomatic left ventricular dysfunction (ejection fraction of < 40 per cent or significant regional wall motion abnormality) should also receive ACE inhibitor.

Warfarin therapy should be considered for patients with extensive anterior infarction. A screening echocardiogram should be carried out, and warfarin commenced in those with high risk of intraventricular thrombus. Treatment should continue for six months. After six months, the risk of an embolic event is reduced (unless there is co-existent AF). Since aspirin is superior to warfarin in the prevention of post-infarct cardiac events, it is reasonable to consider withdrawing warfarin from patients in sinus rhythm who have been treated for six months and replacing it with aspirin.

As well as reducing cholesterol levels, HMG CoA reductase inhibitors have many beneficial effects on the pathological processes involved in coronary artery disease, including improving endothelial function, antiplatelet and anticoagulant effects and prevention of lipoprotein oxidation. These effects will help to stabilize atheromatous plaques and reduce the risk of coronary thrombosis. The role of HMG CoA reductase inhibitors in the secondary prevention of cardiac events following MI has been evaluated in over 17 000 patients randomized in the 4S, CARE and LIPID studies. These studies show that lipid lowering therapy with a statin following a MI reduces the risk of death, recurrent infarction and the need for revascularization procedures by about 25 per cent. Benefit is seen for both men and women, in older subjects, and in those with only moderate hyperlipidaemia. On the basis of these trials, the Standing Medical Advisory Committee of the Department of Health recommends lipid lowering therapy with simvastatin 20 mg daily or pravastatin 40 mg daily for all patients with a cholesterol level of >4.8 mmol/l. The dose of the HMG CoA reductase inhibitor may need to be modified, or the addition of other agents considered in patients with resistant hyperlipidaemia.

Risk stratification

A non-selective strategy of carrying out cardiac catheterization and revascularization in all post-infarct patients does not improve survival. Risk stratification using a combination of clinical predictors and stress testing can identify high risk subgroups who will benefit from catheterization, and help to optimize post-infarction treatment. Patients with high risk clinical features (post-infarction angina, previous infarction, heart failure) who are candidates for revascularization should be referred for early angiography without further investigation, as the risk of a further event or death is high, and their prognosis may be improved by revascularization. Patients who have favourable clinical features (no history of previous infarction and no heart failure) should undergo early stress testing. If available, exercise testing prior to discharge may be useful. A modified Bruce protocol exercise test is safe in the first week post-infarction. Many patients benefit psychologically from an early exercise test, and the data helps to plan an investigation strategy prior to discharge. In many hospitals, limited resources prevent all patients from undergoing in-hospital exercise testing. A symptom-limited Bruce protocol treadmill exercise test can be safely carried out four weeks post-infarction, and the result reviewed at the first outpatient visit, six weeks post-infarction. Exercise tests should be performed without interrupting treatment with beta-blockers. Patients who have low risk features and a negative exercise test have an annual mortality rate of around one per cent and can be managed conservatively. Patients with ST depression at low workload, or an inability to increase their systolic pressure during exercise, usually have extensive coronary disease and/or significantly impaired left ventricular function and an annual mortality rate of around 20 per cent. Cardiac catheterization with a view to revascularization is indicated in these higher risk patients. If a standard exercise treadmill test cannot be completed because of musculoskeletal or respiratory problems, a pharmacological isotope perfusion scan will provide reliable information on the presence of inducible ischaemia.

Patients with late (after the first 24 hours) ventricular arrhythmias are at high risk of sudden cardiac death. They require referral to an electrophysiologist to determine an optimal treatment strategy from the options of revascularization, electrophysiologically guided drug therapy, AICD implantation, and empirical treatment with amiodarone.

Risk stratification and management during the recovery phase of acute myocardial infarction

Key points

- Lifestyle modification and rehabilitation (including smoking cessation) will improve quality of life and prognosis.

- Driving should be prohibited for four weeks and flying for six weeks following an uncomplicated infarct. Patients with complications may need further assessment before being allowed to drive or fly.

- Beta-blockers, aspirin and ACE inhibitors are indicated in a large proportion of patients. An echocardiogram will help to guide prescription of ACE inhibitors and warfarin in some patients.

- All patients with a cholesterol of >4.8 mmol/l should be considered for drug therapy with a HMG CoA reductase inhibitor.

- Exercise testing post-infarction will help to select patients who may benefit from early angiography and revascularization.

- Patients with late ventricular arrhythmias should be reviewed by an electrophysiologist to plan an optimal treatment strategy.

References

Beller, G. A. (1997). Determining prognosis after acute MI in the thrombolytic era. *Br. Med. J.*, **14**, 761–762.

Bethell, H. J. N. (1996). Going home. The first few weeks after a heart attack. *Br. Med. J.*, **312**, 1372–1373.

Burr, M. L., Fehily, A. M., Gilbert, J. F., *et al.* (1989). Effects of changes in fat, fish and fibre intake on death and reinfarction. Diet and reinfarction trial. *Lancet*, **2**, 757–761.

Byrne, C. D. and Wild, S. H. (1996). Lipids and secondary prevention of ischaemic heart disease. *Br. Med. J.*, **313**, 1273–1274.

Cairns, A. J. (1994). Oral anticoagulants or aspirin after MI? *Lancet*, **343**, 497–498.

Chua, T. P. and Lipkin, D. P. (1993). Cardiac rehabilitation. *Br. Med. J.*, **306**, 731–732.

Cooper, A. J. (1985). MI and advice on sexual activity. *Practitioner*, **229**, 575–579.

Daly, L. E., Graham, I. M., Hickey, M., *et al.* (1985). Does stopping smoking delay onset of angina after infarction? *Br. Med. J.*, **291**, 935–937.

Daviglus, M. L., Stamler, J., Greenland, P., *et al.* (1997). Fish consumption and risk of coronary heart disease. What does the evidence show? *Eur. Heart J.*, **18**, 1841–1842.

—99—

Davis, R. M. (1997). Passive smoking: history repeats itself. *Br. Med. J.*, **315**, 961–962.

Doll, R. (1997). One for the heart. *Br. Med. J.*, **315**, 1664–1668.

Felstein, I. (1993). Sex and the heart attack patient. *Br. J. Cardiol.*, **1**, 13.

Flapan, A. D. (1994). Management of patients after their first MI. *Br. Med. J.*, **309**, 1129–1134.

Freeman, I. J., King, J. C. (1986). Sex and the post infarction patient. *Cardiology in Practice*, **14**, 6–8.

Gillman, M. W. (1996). Enjoy your fruits and vegetables. *Br. Med. J.*, **313**, 765–766.

Gohlke, H., Gohlke-Barwolf (1998). Cardiac rehabilitation. *Eur. Heart J.*, **19**, 1004–1010.

Law, M. R., Morris, J. K. and Wald, N. J. (1997). Environmental tobacco smoke exposure and ischaemic heart disease: an evaluation of the evidence. *Br. Med. J.*, **315**, 973–980.

Levy, J. (1994). How to help your patients stop smoking. *Br. J. Cardiol.*, **2**, 77–78.

Lim, R., Kreidieh, I., Dyke, L., *et al.* (1994). Exercise testing without interruption of medication for refining the selection of mildly symptomatic patients for prognostic coronary angiography. *Br. Heart J.*, **71**, 334–340.

Neiderberger, M. (1995). Early exercise testing after MI and thrombolysis. *Eur. Heart J.*, **16**, 1161–1162.

Olsson, G., Odden, A., Johansson, L., *et al.* (1988). Prognosis after withdrawal of chronic post-infarction metoprolol treatment: a two to seven year follow up. *Eur. Heart J.*, **9**, 365–372.

Wilhelmsson, C., Vedin, A., Elmfeldt, D., *et al.* (1975). Smoking and MI. *Lancet*, **1**, 415–420.

Winyard, G. (1997). *SMAC Statement on Use of Statins*. London: Department of Health. (EL (97) 41 HCD IP Aug 97.)

Working Group for the Study of Transdermal Nicotine in Patients with Coronary Artery Disease. (1994). Nicotine replacement therapy for patients with coronary artery disease. *Arch. Intern. Med.*, **154**, 989–995.

16

Non-Q-wave myocardial infarction

Background

Non-Q-wave MI has become more common since the introduction of reperfusion therapy, and now accounts for approximately 30 per cent of all infarctions. Only a quarter of patients with non-Q-wave infarction present with chest pain and ST elevation, and in these patients, early clot lysis limits the extent of myocardial necrosis. The majority of patients who develop non-Q-wave infarction present with unstable angina and ST depression; in these patients intermittent vessel occlusion leads to episodes of limited myocardial necrosis. Irrespective of the initial presentation, these patients have a relatively small rise in cardiac enzymes (usually in the range of 500–1500 IU for CK) with no Q-wave formation on the 12 lead ECG, indicating that only a relatively small infarction has occurred.

The pattern of early mortality and late complications associated with non-Q-wave infarction is very different to that associated with complete Q-wave infarction. During the first weeks after non-Q-wave infarction, early mortality is 50 per cent less than in Q-wave infarction, related to the relatively limited ventricular damage that occurs. In many patients, however, functioning but ischaemic myocardium survives in the territory supplied by the diseased artery that caused the initial presentation. The presence of this residual ischaemia results in a high rate of angina and early reinfarction, and the mortality rate after two years is identical to that associated with an initially more extensive Q-wave infarction.

Management

Management strategies for patients with non-Q-wave MI have been evaluated in almost 1500 patients randomized in the TIMI IIIB and recently reported VANQWISH studies. These studies compared a strategy of early angiography and revascularization for all patients with a strategy of medical therapy with angiography and revascularization for only those patients with refractory symptoms or an early positive pre-discharge stress test. The strategy of early non-selective intervention had no beneficial effect on long-term mortality, and was associated with a high complication rate. The use of diltiazem to prevent reinfarction in non-Q-wave infarction was examined in the MDPIT study. Patients randomized to diltiazem had a lower reinfarction rate during follow up, although the statistical power of the study was limited. Taking this data into account, we currently recommend that:

1. All patients with non-Q-wave infarction should optimally be treated with a beta-blocker and aspirin. Risk factor management should be optimized.

2. Diltiazem 60–120 mg tds can be added for patients with good left ventricular function, and may reduce the subsequent reinfarction rate.

3. Patients who have recurrent ischaemia during their hospital stay should be considered for angiography and revascularization.

4. Patients who settle on medical therapy should optimally have a pre-discharge symptom-limited exercise test. Patients with an early positive test should also be considered for angiography and revascularization.

Patients whose symptoms settle on medical therapy and who have a satisfactory stress test can be managed with continuing medical therapy.

Key points

- Non-Q-wave infarction has become more common since the introduction of thrombolytic therapy and improved treatment of unstable angina.

- The occurrence of significant residual ischaemia in many patients leads to a high incidence of post-infarction angina and reinfarction.

- Diltiazem may reduce the early reinfarction rate and should be prescribed to patients with a modest enzyme rise but no Q-wave formation, if left ventricular function is good.

- High risk patients should be considered for cardiac catheterization as an inpatient, with PTCA or referral for CABG as appropriate.

References

Gibson, R. S., Boden, W. E., Theroux, P., *et al.* (1986). Diltiazem and reinfarction in patients with non-Q-wave infarction. *N. Engl. J. Med.*, **315**, 423–429.

TIMI IIIB investigators. (1994). Effects of tissue plasminogen activator and comparison of early invasive and conservative strategies in unstable angina and non-Q-wave MI. *Circulation*, **89**, 1545–1556.

Wong, S. C., Greenberg, H., Hager, W. D., *et al.* (1992). Effect of diltiazem on recurrent MI in patients with non-Q-wave MI. *J. Am. Coll. Cardiol.*, **19**, 1421–1425.

17   Unstable angina

Background

Unstable angina, defined simply as new onset angina or angina that is increasing in frequency, severity or duration, is a common clinical syndrome with a relatively poor prognosis which affects around 300 000 people in the UK each year. In the year following an episode of unstable angina, as many as 15 per cent of patients will die or suffer an MI, and a further 15 per cent will require a revascularization procedure. Most of these events occur within three months of the episode in easily identified high risk patients.

The pathophysiology underlying unstable angina has been well described. Rupture of an atheromatous plaque initiates activation of platelets and the coagulation cascade, leading to the formation of a thrombus which partially occludes the vessel lumen, limiting blood flow with resultant myocardial ischaemia. Plaques at increased risk of rupture are eccentric and lipid rich, with evidence of active inflammation. Plaque rupture and thrombus formation occur when vulnerable lesions are subjected to stress forces associated with fluctuations in blood pressure and coronary artery tone in the presence of adverse changes in platelet or coagulation activity. Factors such as physical exertion, smoking, diet and diurnal variation in endogenous coagulation activity are therefore important in initiating episodes of unstable angina. Following plaque disruption it can take up to three months for a lesion to heal and re-endothelialize, providing a potential site capable of initiating further unstable episodes over this time period.

Our understanding of the pathophysiology of unstable angina has helped to develop rational treatment strategies aimed at controlling symptoms and improving prognosis. Antiplatelet therapy with aspirin has shown beneficial effects in four randomized placebo-controlled studies, with an approximate 50 per cent reduction in the rate of death or MI that is maintained for at least two years. The first dose should be a minimum of 300 mg of a rapidly absorbed formulation, followed by a maintenance dose of 75 mg daily. Studies suggest that continuous intravenous infusion of unfractionated heparin commenced early in the course of unstable angina and given in doses sufficient to maintain the APTT between two and three times control, will significantly reduce the rate of death or MI during hospitalization. A combination of aspirin and heparin is more effective than either agent alone. Conventional heparin therapy has a substantial failure rate, probably related to the unpredictable anti-coagulant response to intravenous unfractionated heparin, as well as its neutralization by protein binding and activated platelets. Low molecular weight heparin (LMWH) has a more predictable anticoagulant effect, and does not therefore require monitoring of the APTT, has improved antithrombolitic efficacy, and is resistant to inhibition by activated platelets. In the FRISC, FRIC and ESSENCE studies, use of LMWH in unstable angina was investigated in over 6000 patients. The data from these studies shows that:

1. LMWH is superior to placebo (63 per cent reduction in death and myocardial infarction in FRISC)

2. LMWH is at least as effective as intravenous heparin (FRIC study), and may reduce the rate of short-term (30 day) cardiac events by around 15 per cent compared to intravenous unfractionated heparin (ESSENCE study), with no increase in the risk of major bleeding. The difference in the results obtained in the ESSENCE study compared to those from the FRIC study may relate to a superior anticoagulant profile of the LMWH used in ESSENCE. These studies support a change from intravenous heparin to subcutaneous LMWH, given for one week.

The increased initial cost of LMWH compared to intravenous heparin is offset by reduced in-hospital patient costs related to the lower event rate associated with LMWH. In the FRISC study, longer term LMWH was not beneficial in the prevention of late cardiac events, but the dosing regime used may have been sub-optimal. The important question of longer term use of higher dose LMWH following an episode of unstable angina will be evaluated in over 3000 patients enrolled in the FRISC II trial.

Beta-blockers reduce myocardial oxygen consumption in patients with unstable angina. The pooled results of three randomized controlled trials suggest that beta-blockers reduce the rate of MI by around 10 per cent, and they should be prescribed for all patients, unless a contraindication is present. If a beta-blocker is contraindicated, and left ventricular function is good, a calcium antagonist with additional heart rate slowing effects (such as diltiazem or verapamil) is an alternative. In patients with unstable angina and impaired left ventricular function, calcium antagonists (particularly dihydropyridine agents such as nifedipine) should be avoided.

Intravenous nitrates reduce myocardial oxygen consumption by systemic vasodilation, increase collateral flow to ischaemic areas by coronary vasodilation, and have an additional antiplatelet effect. Tolerance to intravenous nitrates develops rapidly, and the use of interrupted oral regimes that allow a nitrate-free interval may be preferable after the first 24 hours of therapy.

Although thrombus formation is important in the pathophysiology of unstable angina, a number of small studies and meta-analysis of the MI trials show no beneficial effect for thrombolytic therapy in the treatment of unstable angina. This may be due to adverse platelet activation induced by thrombolytic agents offsetting beneficial effects on clot lysis. Thrombolytic therapy should only be given to patients who progress from unstable angina to acute MI associated with ST elevation or new bundle branch block.

Recently, data on almost 5000 patients with unstable angina randomized to standard therapy or standard therapy plus additional antiplatelet therapy with a glycoprotein IIb/IIIa inhibitor in the PRISM studies has provisionally been reported. Additional therapy with a glycoprotein IIb/IIIa inhibitor reduced death, MI and recurrent ischaemia by around 30 per cent. Although these agents do not currently have a licence for use in unstable angina, it is likely that they will become widely used if further studies confirm these promising results. Initial reports of studies evaluating direct thrombin inhibitors such as hirudin in the treatment of unstable angina have been less promising, and these agents may have little clinical advantage over therapy with LMWH.

Management of recent onset or worsening angina

Patients with recent onset of exertional angina or those with worsening angina who have not had severe, prolonged or rest pain in the last two weeks and who have no new ST or T-wave changes on their resting ECG are at low risk of death or MI. These patients do not require admission to hospital. Patients with new onset symptoms should be commenced on aspirin and a beta-blocker, and drug therapy should be increased in those with deteriorating symptoms. An early outpatient appointment in the cardiology department to facilitate assessment of the response to the initiation or change in therapy should be arranged. Patients who do not respond to the introduction or modification of medical therapy should be considered for exercise testing or angiography to assess their suitability for revascularization.

Management of patients with ischaemic chest pain at rest

All patients who have an episode of ischaemic chest pain at rest that is not easily attributable to an external factor such as emotional stress or exposure to low temperature should be admitted to hospital, ideally to CCU. The presence of ECG abnormalities on the admission ECG (ST depression, or T-wave inversion), particularly if they occur in association with pain, increase the likelihood of significant underlying ischaemic heart disease as a cause of the patient's chest pain. A normal ECG, however, does not exclude the diagnosis. Where diagnostic doubt exists in a patient with episodes of chest pain at rest, it is appropriate to admit the patient for treatment and investigation with a diagnosis of possible unstable angina and await the results of subsequent investigations before arriving at a definitive diagnosis. Patients with high risk features should have high priority for admission to CCU if bed availability is limited. Initial investigation and treatment consists of the following:

1. Check blood count, electrolytes, glucose and cholesterol, and arrange a cardiac enzyme and ECG series. Institute continuous ST segment monitoring if available, or obtain a 12 lead ECG with any episodes of recurrent chest pain.

2. Treat any exacerbating conditions such as anaemia or heart failure, and correct hyperglycaemia with IV insulin if glucose >11 mmol/l.

3. Commence aspirin 300 mg orally followed by 75 mg daily long-term.

4. Commence enoxaparin 1 mg/kg bd subcutaneously.

5. Commence metoprolol 50 mg bd, with the dose increased as necessary to achieve a resting heart rate of 50–60 bpm. If a beta-blocker is contraindicated and left ventricular function is good, give diltiazem 60–180 mg tds.

6. Commence low dose intravenous nitrates for 24 hours, switching to a once daily oral preparation after this.

There is no evidence that routine cardiac catheterization and revascularization of all patients with unstable angina improves prognosis, although the TIMI-IIIb study suggests that this strategy shortens hospital stay.

Patients should be classified into a low risk subgroup who can be safely managed medically, and a high risk subgroup who may require catheterization and revascularization as inpatients.

Risk stratification and further management

Low risk patients

Patients with no previous history of ischaemic heart disease whose symptoms settle with the above treatment regime, who have normal cardiac enzymes and do not have ECG, haemodynamic or rhythm changes in association with episodes of pain, are at low risk of early death or MI. In these patients, switch from intravenous to oral nitrates after 24 hours and mobilize the patient. Continue with subcutaneous heparin for 3–7 days.

The patient's risk factor profile should be optimized, with advice on lifestyle, smoking and treatment of hyperlipidaemia with a statin if cholesterol >4.8 mmol/l. Optimally, in patients who are candidates for revascularization, a stress test should be carried out when the patient has been free of episodes of ischaemia for a minimum period of 48 hours. Patients with an early positive stress test should be considered for angiography to help determine their optimal treatment strategy (see next section for guidelines based on angiographic findings). Patients with a negative stress test or who are unsuitable for revascularization should be discharged after a minimum of 48 hours with stable symptoms, and their progress reviewed in the outpatient clinic within six weeks. The cardiac event rate in low risk patients with a negative stress test in the six months following an episode of unstable angina is less than five per cent

High risk patients

Patients with any of the following features are at increased risk of early death or MI:

1. Recurrent episodes of ischaemic chest pain at rest, particularly if associated with reversible ST depression
2. Previous history of MI or prior revascularization procedure
3. Clinical evidence of haemodynamic compromise (hypotension, pulmonary oedema or transient mitral regurgitation) in association with episodes of ischaemia
4. Episodes of ventricular tachycardia
5. Early positive stress test

6. Small increase in cardiac enzymes, associated with the occurrence of minimal myocardial damage. Conventional biochemical measures of myocardial necrosis such as CK levels are abnormal in only five per cent of patients with unstable angina. Around 30 per cent of patients with unstable angina, however, have evidence of minimal myocardial damage if more sensitive markers such as cardiac troponin T or troponin I are used.

The cardiac event rate in the six months after an episode of unstable angina in patients with any of the above six features is approximately 30 per cent. Recurrent episodes of ischaemia should be treated by intensifying the medical regime (if blood pressure is >100 mmHg, increase the intravenous nitrate infusion rate, ensure heart rate is maintained in range of 50–60 bpm by increasing dose of beta-blocker or adding diltiazem 60–180 mg tds, give appropriate treatment for rhythm disturbances or heart failure and treat persistent pain with intravenous diamorphine).

Patients with high risk features should be considered for inpatient cardiac catheterization to determine whether revascularization is possible. The optimal time to schedule catheterization in these patients has not yet been determined. The complications rate for coronary angioplasty in patients with unstable angina is reduced by a period of heparin therapy prior to the procedure, and it is therefore reasonable to attempt to stabilize high risk patients medically, and defer catheterization for 72 hours. Patients who are highly unstable with frequent episodes of ischaemia that persist despite maximal medical therapy may require earlier investigation; in these patients insertion of an intra-aortic balloon pump, if available, may help to stabilize the patient prior to the catheterization. In these high risk patients, administration of a IIa/IIIb inhibitor will reduce PTCA complication rates by about one third.

The subsequent management of high risk patients depends on the findings at cardiac catheterization. Patients with three vessel disease or left main stem stenosis will benefit symptomatically and prognostically from coronary bypass surgery. In patients with one or two vessel disease, coronary angioplasty with dilatation of the culprit lesion implicated by the distribution of ECG changes is safe and effective.

Key points

- Unstable angina is common, and patients have a high risk of death or MI or the need for coronary revascularization. The risk is at a maximum during the three months following the episode of unstable angina.

- Recent studies indicate that aspirin is effective at reducing event rate by 50 per cent, and that LMWH is at least as good as IV heparin.

- Patients with recent onset or worsening angina and no resting ischaemia can be managed with medical therapy and early outpatient follow up.

- Patients with ischaemic chest pain at rest require hospital admission and treatment with aspirin, LMWH, beta-blockers and IV nitrates.

- Patients with high risk features should be considered for cardiac catheterization as inpatients, preferably after 72 hours of intensive medical therapy, with angioplasty or referral for coronary grafting depending on the distribution of coronary disease.

- Low risk patients can be discharged after 48–72 hours of clinical stability, and have a low (five per cent) event rate over the following six months.

References

Antiplatelet Trialists' Collaboration. (1994). Collaborative overview of randomized trials of antiplatelet therapy (Part 1). Prevention of death, prolonged antiplatelet therapy in various categories of patients. *Br. Med. J.*, **308**, 81–106.

Armstrong, P. W. (1997). Heparin in acute coronary disease – requiem for a heavyweight? *N. Engl. J. Med.*, **337**, 492–494.

Braunwald, E., Jones, R. H., Mark, D. B., *et al.* (1994). Diagnosing and managing unstable angina. *Circulation*, **90**, 613–622.

Fox, K. A. A. and Bosanquet, N. (1998). Assessing the UK cost implications of the use of low molecular weight heparin in unstable coronary artery disease. *Br. J. Cardiol.*, **5**, 92–105.

Hamm, C. N., Goldmann, B. U., Heeschen, C., *et al.* (1997). Emergency room triage of patients with acute chest pain by means of rapid testing for cardiac troponin T or troponin I. *N. Eng. J. Med.*, **337**, 1648–1653.

McMurray, J. and Rankin, A. (1994). Cardiology – 1: Treatment of MI, unstable angina and angina pectoris. *Br. Med. J.*, **304**, 1343–1350.

Meinertz, T. and Hamm, C. W. (1998). Rapid testing for cardiac troponins in patients with acute chest pain in the emergency room. *Eur. Heart J.*, **19**, 973–974.

Pitt, B. (1996). Risk stratification in patients with unstable angina. *Circulation*, **93**, 1618–1620.

Rodak, D. J. and Gersh, B. J. (1997). Parallel testing: is it 'T-time'? *Eur. Heart J.*, **18**, 716–718.

Sharma, G. V. R. K., Deupree, R. H., Luchi, R. J., *et al.* (1994). Identification of unstable angina patients who have favourable outcome with medical or surgical therapy (eight year follow up of the Veterans Administration Co-operative Study). *Am. J. Cardiol.*, **74**, 454–458.

Teo, K. K. (1998). Recent advances in cardiology. *Br. Med. J.*, **316**, 911–915.

18

Common arrhythmias not associated with acute myocardial infarction

Background

Cardiac arrhythmias are a common cause of symptoms in patients presenting as emergency medical attendances. In many patients, these will be clearly associated with the symptoms and signs of acute MI, and their treatment is detailed in Chapter 8. This chapter deals with arrhythmias that occur in patients with other cardiovascular and medical disorders. Optimal treatment of these patients depends on establishing the correct diagnosis, initially by clinical assessment and analysis of the 12 lead ECG. In the emergency treatment of tachyarrhythmias, it is better to become familiar with the use of a small number of antiarrhythmic agents. The vast majority of tachyarrhythmias that are not related to an MI can be treated with adenosine, lignocaine or amiodarone, and other drugs are rarely needed. If treatment with these first line agents is ineffective, consult a senior colleague, as polypharmacy can be dangerous. In the treatment of bradyarrhythmias, the insertion of temporary pacing wires can be associated with major complications (particularly if the operator is inexperienced), and many patients are best dealt with initially by observation.

Supraventricular tachyarrhythmias

Supraventricular tachyarrhythmias arise from above the level of the bundle of His. Since ventricular activation occurs via the normal conduction system, the QRS complexes will be narrow in the majority of patients with a supraventricular tachyarrhythmia (although a broad complex configuration can occur if there is pre-existing or rate related bundle branch block or an accessory pathway). Supraventricular tachyarrhythmias can arise from the atrial myocardium (AF, atrial flutter and atrial tachycardia), the region of the atrioventricular junction (atrioventricular nodal re-entry tachycardia – AVNRT) or involve an accessory pathway (atrioventricular re-entry tachycardia). Atrial fibrillation, atrial flutter, AVNRT and atrioventricular re-entry tachycardia are relatively common, whereas atrial tachycardias are rare.

Atrial fibrillation

Atrial fibrillation is the commonest atrial tachyarrhythmia, and occurs more frequently in older patients (AF is present in 0.5 per cent of people under the age of 60 years, and 10 per cent of people over the age of 70 years). In patients who have not had a recent MI, new onset AF usually arises as a complication of atrial distention due to mitral valve disease, hypertensive heart disease, impaired left ventricular function of any aetiology, pulmonary embolism, cor-pulmonale or intracardiac shunts. Other less common causes of AF are cardiac trauma (including cardiac surgery), metabolic abnormalities (such as thyrotoxicosis), exposure to toxins (such as alcohol), pericardial disease or as a non-specific response to infection, all of which can affect the electrical properties of the atrial myocardium. In some patients, AF can arise in an otherwise entirely normal heart.

Regardless of the underlying aetiology, patients with AF develop multiple random wavelets of depolarization in the atrial myocardium, leading to chaotic disorganized atrial depolarization. The atrioventricular node is constantly bombarded with rapid erratic electrical impulses, which are intermittently conducted to the ventricles. Recent onset AF is often associated with palpitations due to the erratic and rapid ventricular rhythm. Heart failure may occur, particularly in patients with coexistent valvular heart disease or impaired left ventricular function. The combination of a rapid ventricular rate and loss of co-ordinated atrial mechanical activity may be associated with a fall in cardiac output of up to 50 per cent. In patients in whom AF persists for more than 48 hours, stasis of blood in the fibrillating atrium may lead to clot formation and systemic embolism.

As noted in Chapter 8, the 12 lead ECG of patients with AF will show an absence of P-waves, erratic fibrillation activity visible in the baseline between ventricular complexes, and an unevenly irregular ventricular rhythm with narrow QRS complexes (unless pre-existing bundle branch block, rate related bundle branch block or an accessory pathway is present). The ventricular rate is usually rapid in untreated patients.

The treatment of recent onset AF depends on the associated symptoms and degree of haemodynamic disturbance. The majority of patients with recent onset AF should receive treatment aimed at restoring sinus rhythm, thereby maintaining optimal cardiac function and avoiding the risk of thromboembolism. Patients who present with recent onset AF should have a full clinical assessment (including a 12 lead ECG, CXR and echocardiogram, if possible) to establish the degree of haemodynamic disturbance present, look for underlying aetiological factors, and determine the length of time since the onset of the arrhythmia. The treatment of AF associated acute MI is dealt with in Chapter 8. In patients with recent onset AF associated with the conditions listed above, treatment is as follows:

1. Institute treatment for obvious precipitating or associated problems such as heart failure, airways disease, pulmonary embolism or thyrotoxicosis. Withdraw precipitants such as alcohol. Check electrolytes and correct hypokalaemia if present.

2. If the AF is poorly tolerated or associated with adverse haemodynamic features (rate >200 bpm, systolic BP <90 mmHg), urgent DC cardioversion is indicated.

3. If the AF has been present for >24 hours or it is impossible to establish the duration of the arrhythmia, early elective cardioversion carries an unacceptably high risk of thromboembolism. In patients with significant mitral valve disease or marked left atrial enlargement, it is unlikely that stable sinus rhythm will be achieved or maintained. Patients in these two groups should be established on oral anticoagulants, and the ventricular rate controlled (aiming for a resting rate of 90 bpm) with digoxin. After one month's stable oral anticoagulant therapy, elective DC cardioversion should be considered in selected patients.

4. If the duration of AF is <24 hours and the arrhythmia is well tolerated, attempted pharmacological cardioversion is indicated. Digoxin may prolong the duration of episodes of AF (it has a pro-arrhythmic effect on atrial myocardium), and is ineffective at rapidly controlling ventricular rate (since its AV nodal blocking effect may be negated in patients with acute symptoms and high sympathetic activity). A number of Class III antiarrhythmic agents are efficacious in rapidly restoring sinus rhythm. Since IV amiodarone produces rapid slowing of the ventricular rate, induces early reversion to sinus rhythm in the majority of patients and is safe and well tolerated even in patients with left ventricular dysfunction, it is our first choice drug for the treatment of recent onset AF. For appropriate patients, commence treatment with amiodarone IV as detailed in Chapter 24. Heparin should be commenced at the same time, and anticoagulation with warfarin instituted for at least one month to minimize the risk of embolization following reversion to sinus rhythm for at least one month. If reversion to sinus rhythm does

not occur within 48 hours of the onset of the arrhythmia, commence oral digoxin and anticoagulants and consider elective cardioversion after one month of treatment.

Atrial flutter

Atrial flutter is much less common than AF, and is almost always associated with underlying significant cardiac abnormalities such as mitral valve disease or ischaemic heart disease with left ventricular dysfunction, leading to atrial enlargement. In typical atrial flutter, an organized circular re-entry circuit depolarizes in an anticlockwise direction down the lateral border of the right atrium and back up the intra-atrial septum, at a rate of 300 per minute. The normal AV node cannot conduct at this rate, and 2:1 atrioventricular block usually occurs. The 12 lead ECG shows a regular narrow complex tachycardia (unless there is pre-existing or a rate related bundle branch block) at a rate of 150 bpm with saw tooth flutter waves visible between the QRS complexes (usually best seen in V1) (Figure 18.1). Atrial flutter may be associated with palpitations or haemodynamic compromise, due to the rapid ventricular rate and loss of effective atrial mechanical activity. If you are unsure whether a tachycardia is due to atrial flutter, vagal manoeuvres (such as carotid sinus massage) or a bolus of intravenous adenosine will temporarily increase the degree of atrioventricular block present, reveal the characteristic flutter waves, and allow an accurate diagnosis to be made (Figure 18.2). Treatment of atrial flutter depends on the clinical circumstances; e.g.:

1. If the arrhythmia is associated with significant haemodynamic compromise (systolic BP < 90 mmHg), or symptoms of angina, impaired conscious level or heart failure, urgent DC cardioversion is the treatment of choice.

2. If the arrhythmia is well tolerated, an attempt can be made to control it with drug therapy. Atrial flutter is often resistant to treatment with drugs. Class I antiarrhythmic drugs may terminate atrial flutter, but can also cause a poorly tolerated increase in ventricular rate (by slowing the flutter rate to less than 300 per minute and therefore facilitating 1:1 atrioventricular conduction at a rate greater than 150 bpm). Amiodarone has beneficial effects on atrial electrical stability, and may terminate the arrhythmia. In addition amiodarone impairs atrioventricular conduction, and this property will help to slow the ventricular rate. We therefore recommend IV amiodarone for the treatment of atrial flutter, using the regime detailed in Chapter 24. Although atrial flutter is a relatively organized rhythm and thrombus formation is less likely to occur, anticoagulation should not be used as in atrial fibrillation, particularly if other risk factors (such as marked atrial enlargement or mitral valve disease) are present.

3. Overdrive pacing is an alternative treatment that is effective in restoring

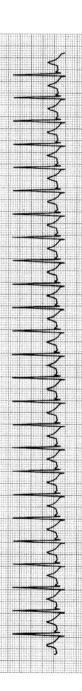

Figure 18.1 Regular narrow complex tachycardia with a rate of 150 bpm in a patient with atrial flutter.

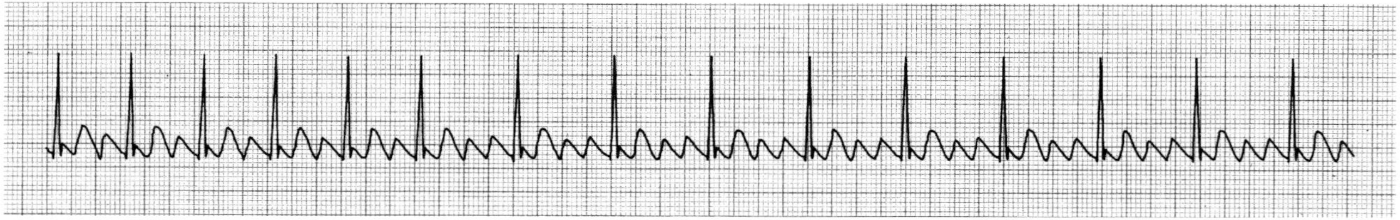

Figure 18.2 The response of atrial flutter to temporary AV nodal blockade induced by IV adenosine. Ventricular rate is temporarily slowed to 75 bpm, revealing underlying atrial flutter waves with a rate of 300 bpm.

sinus rhythm in 70 per cent of patients. If facilities are available, position a temporary pacing wire against the lateral wall of the right atrium. A burst of rapid atrial pacing at a rate of 400 bpm for several seconds will usually restore sinus rhythm. Occasionally AF will be precipitated, and this will often spontaneously revert to sinus rhythm. If it persists, it is easier to treat than atrial flutter.

4. If atrial flutter persists despite 24 hours of intravenous amiodarone, or is resistant to overdrive pacing, DC cardioversion (often at very low energies) has a high success rate in restoring sinus rhythm.

Atrioventricular nodal re-entry tachycardia

Atrioventricular nodal re-entry is the mechanism present in 70 per cent of patients with paroxysmal regular supraventricular tachycardia. Symptoms can develop at any time, but are most common in women aged between 30 and 50 years. Patients with the common form of AVNRT have two or more functional pathways with differing conduction rates within the atrioventricular node. An atrial ectopic beat that occurs at an appropriate time is conducted from atria to ventricles via one nodal pathway, returns immediately to the atria via the other pathway, and continuously re-initiates the cycle. Patients with AVNRT have structurally normal hearts, and the arrhythmia is not life-threatening. In the majority of patients the characteristics of the nodal re-entry circuit lead to the atria and ventricles being depolarized simultaneously, and the resultant P-waves are superimposed on the QRS complex and are therefore rarely visible. Inspection of the 12 lead ECG during the common form of AVNRT will show a rapid regular narrow complex tachycardia (rate 150–250 bpm) with no visible P-waves (Figure 18.3). If P-waves are visible between the QRS complexes, it implies that the arrhythmia has a mechanism other than common AVNRT. The tachycardia can induce ST segment and T-wave changes that persist for some time after the cessation of the arrhythmia, but these are of no significance. The ECG during sinus rhythm is normal.

In rare instances of severe haemodynamic deterioration with AVNRT, immediate DC cardioversion should be performed. Most tachycardias are, however, well tolerated and vagal manoeuvres (carotid sinus massage, Valsalva manoeuvre or application of cold water to the face) should be tried initially. If vagal manoeuvres fail, drug therapy is indicated.

First line drug therapy is adenosine, which is effective in terminating the vast majority of episodes of AVNRT. It has a very short half-life of 5–10 seconds, and causes no significant haemodynamic side-effects. Transient

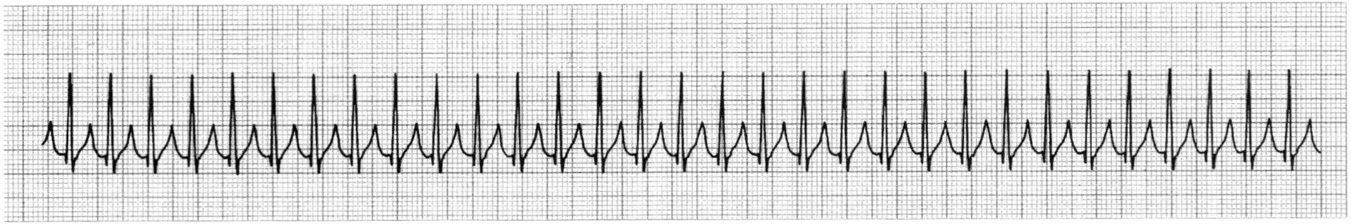

Figure 18.3 AVNRT. Rapid (190 bpm) regular complex tachycardia. No P-waves visible between QRS complexes.

facial flushing, dyspnoea and chest pain are common, but last for less than 20 seconds. Adenosine is given as a rapid IV bolus into a peripheral vein and flushed through with 10 ml of saline, as detailed in Chapter 24. A rhythm strip should be recorded during the administration, as this may aid in defining the nature of the arrhythmia.

Adenosine is contraindicated in patients with asthma or AV block, and should be used with caution in patients with COAD, as bronchospasm may be exacerbated. If bronchospasm occurs, withhold further adenosine and treat with nebulized bronchodilators. Dipyridamole potentiates the effect of adenosine, and dosage should be reduced to an initial 1 mg bolus, increasing to 2 mg and 4 mg in total. Theophyllines antagonize the action of adenosine, and patients receiving such drugs may therefore be resistant to its action.

If adenosine is contraindicated or ineffective, verapamil is an alternative agent effective in the treatment of AVNRT. Verapamil should not be given under the following circumstances:

1. Systolic BP <100 mmHg

2. Patient has known impaired LV function

3. QRS complex duration >120 ms (three small squares)

4. Patient is receiving concurrent treatment with beta-blockers

5. Patient is known to have an accessory pathway.

Verapamil is given as an IV bolus, as detailed in Chapter 24.

If first line drug therapy with adenosine or verapamil fails, the addition of further drugs should be avoided as effects can be unpredictable. In this situation contact a senior colleague, as the tachycardia can usually be terminated by atrial pacing.

To terminate AVNRT by atrial pacing:

1. Place a temporary pacing wire in contact with the endocardium of the right atrium.

2. Attempt to terminate the arrhythmia initially with underdrive pacing; pace the atrium at 100 bpm. If a pacing spike occurs at an appropriate phase of the cardiac cycle, it will render one limb of the re-entry circuit refractory and terminate the arrhythmia.

3. If underdrive pacing fails, attempt overdrive pacing by pacing the right atrium at a rate 20 per cent faster than the tachycardia rate for 30 seconds. On abrupt termination of pacing, sinus rhythm will often resume.

4. More sophisticated methods of tachycardia termination require the

introduction of timed extra stimuli with a programmable stimulator, and are less simple to apply.

If drug therapy and pacing fail to terminate a prolonged symptomatic AVNRT, elective cardioversion is indicated.

Prophylaxis against recurrent attacks of AVNRT is not needed unless attacks are frequent. If symptoms are troublesome, sotalol 40–80 mg tds, verapamil 40–120 mg tds or flecanide 50–200 mg bd (in patients with structurally normal hearts) may be effective. If symptoms are resistant to drug therapy with atrioventricular nodal blocking agents, or if intolerable side-effects occur, referral for radio frequency ablation is preferable to the cumulative risks associated with the use of long-term therapy with Class I or Class III agents.

Supraventricular arrhythmias associated with accessory pathways

In the normal heart, atrial impulses can only be conducted to the ventricles via the AV node. If an accessory pathway exists connecting the atria and ventricle it can act as a mechanism for the generation of rhythm disturbances, and symptomatic supraventricular tachyarrhythmias occur. Accessory pathways can arise in a number of different sites, and connect to a variety of different areas of the atrium, ventricles or conducting system. The surface ECG and characteristic arrhythmias depend on the precise connections and conduction characteristics of the pathway. The presence of an accessory pathway is the mechanism responsible in approximately 20 per cent of patients with symptomatic paroxysmal regular supraventricular tachycardia.

The most common situation arises when an accessory pathway connects atrial and ventricular myocardium. The pathway (Bundle of Kent) is congenital, and can lie anywhere in the AV groove. If the accessory pathway is capable of conduction from atria to ventricles (some pathways will only conduct from ventricle to atria), the surface ECG will show a short PR interval with a broad QRS complex showing an initial delta-wave, due to pre-excitation of the ventricles via the accessory pathway (Figure 18.4). If the delta-wave is positive in lead V1, the pathway is left-sided; if the delta-wave is negative in V1, the pathway is right-sided. More precise location of pathways from the surface ECG is possible, but complex.

Electrocardiographic evidence of an accessory pathway is present in 0.15 per cent of the population, but around 50% of these patients will develop symptomatic arrhythmias. All patients with evidence of an accessory pathway should be assessed by an electrophysiologist to

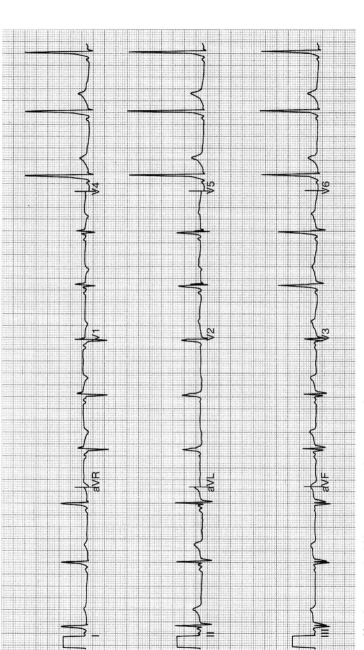

Figure 18.4 Short PR interval and delta-wave in patient with an accessory pathway.

quantify their risk of sudden cardiac death. Sudden cardiac death may occur in patients who have a pathway capable of rapid conduction from atria to ventricles. If AF occurs in these patients, rapid stimulation of the ventricles can result in VF. Patients whose pre-excitation is intermittent or disappears during exercise are unlikely to have a pathway capable of rapid conduction, but the most reliable method of determining the conduction characteristics of the pathway (and therefore defining the risk of sudden cardiac death) is by electrophysiological study (EPS). All patients with evidence of an accessory pathway should therefore be referred to an electrophysiologist for consideration of EPS and possible ablation. The risks of long-term drug therapy for symptomatic arrhythmias are probably greater than the risks of ablation.

The commonest arrhythmia in patients with Wolff–Parkinson–White syndrome (WPW) is atrioventricular re-entry tachycardia (AVRT). The usual form of AVRT occurs when an ectopic initiates a re-entry cycle with impulses passing down the AV node and back up the accessory pathway (orthodromic tachycardia). Since the ventricles are depolarized via the normal conduction system, QRS complexes will be narrow. Atrial activation is delayed until impulses have passed back up to the accessory pathway, and P-waves may therefore be visible between the QRS complexes. The majority of patients with WPW therefore present with an abnormal resting ECG and episodes of symptomatic paroxysmal narrow complex tachycardia. The ECG during tachycardia characteristically shows regular narrow complex tachycardia with P-waves visible between the QRS complexes. QRS alternans may be present in some patients with AVRT. Attacks of paroxysmal narrow complex AVRT in patients with known WPW should be treated with IV Amiodarone, which will interrupt conduction in the accessory pathway. AV nodal blocking agents may precipitate rapid AF, and should be avoided in patients with known WPW.

Atrial fibrillation is less common in patients with WPW, but may be life-threatening. The ECG in AF associated with WPW characteristically shows a rapid and completely irregular ventricular rhythm. Conduction of atrial impulses occurs via both the AV node and the accessory pathway. The morphology of QRS complexes therefore varies from beat to beat, with some complexes showing a broad pre-exciting configuration, while those conducted via the AV node show a normal narrow complex morphology. If rapid AF associated with haemodynamic compromise occurs, proceed directly to DC cardioversion. If the AF is well tolerated, drugs that slow conduction in the accessory pathway should be tried.

A rare form of AVRT can occur in patients with WPW when atrial impulses are conducted down the accessory pathway and back to the atria via the AV node. Since ventricular activation occurs via the accessory pathway, the resultant QRS complexes are pre-excited and the patient presents with a broad complex tachycardia. This is difficult to differentiate from VT or from other aberrantly conducted supraventricular arrhythmias without the aid of EPS.

If a patient with WPW presents with AVRT or AF and haemodynamic compromise, do not give any antiarrhythmic drugs, as they may further depress cardiac output or blood pressure leading to acceleration of the tachycardia (which may then deteriorate into VF). If the tachycardia is well tolerated, initial drug therapy is appropriate. As a general rule, AV nodal blocking drugs should be avoided, as they can have unpredictable deleterious effects (Adverse events with Digoxin and Verapamil have been well documented; more recently there have been reports of rapid unstable AF, precipitated by Adenosine). Drugs such as Flecainide or Amiodarone slow conduction in both the AV node and accessory pathway, and may be preferable for the acute termination of WPW related tachyarrhythmias, but you should always consult a senior colleague prior to their administration. If haemodynamic deterioration occurs during or after the administration of any antiarrhythmic drug, proceed immediately to DC cardioversion.

Other, less common, anatomically and functionally distinct accessory pathways may be associated with arrhythmias. In some patients, a pathway exists which connects atrial and ventricular myocardium but is only able to conduct from ventricle to atria. In normal sinus rhythm, impulses cannot be conducted down the pathway and must be conducted via the normal AV node. The resting surface ECG is therefore normal, and the patient has a concealed pathway. The pathway, however, acts as the substrate for symptomatic re-entry arrhythmias, with impulses passing down the AV node and back up the pathway. The ECG during tachycardia shows a narrow QRS complex. Since atrial activation occurs after ventricular activation via the accessory pathway, a P-wave should be visible following the QRS complex. Patients suspected of having a concealed accessory pathway on the basis of the 12 lead ECG should undergo EPS with a view to ablation. Concealed accessory pathways account for around 20 per cent of paroxysmal regular supraventricular tachycardias. Other pathways can connect parts of the conduction system to the ventricular myocardium. Ventricular activation occurs via the pathway, and the QRS complex has a bundle branch block morphology (usually with a normal PR interval). These patients require full EPS to evaluate the mechanism of their tachycardias. In some patients the accessory pathway accelerates conduction within the AV node (James fibres), with a resultant short PR interval and normal QRS morphology (Lown–Ganong–Levine syndrome). These patients have a tendency to develop re-entrant supraventricular tachyarrhythmias (occurring in 10 per cent of such patients), and usually respond to conventional treatment with adenosine.

Ectopic atrial tachycardia

Unifocal atrial tachycardia arises from a single area of myocardium outside the sinus node but within the left or right atrium, and accounts for 5–10 per cent of patients with symptomatic paroxysmal supraventricular tachycardia. In this arrhythmia, the atrial rate is usually less than 250 bpm. Each QRS complex is preceded by a morphologically abnormal P-wave (the precise configuration of the P-wave depends on the site of origin of the ectopic focus). Since unifocal atrial tachycardia is not dependent on a circuit involving the atrioventricular node, nodal blockade with calcium antagonists or beta-blockade will not terminate the arrhythmia but may slow the ventricular rate. Attacks may be prevented by atrial membrane stabilizing drugs such as sotalol. Since this arrhythmia is difficult to treat, seek the advice of an electrophysiologist if suggestive features of atrial tachycardia are present on the 12 lead ECG.

Unifocal atrial tachycardia may arise as a complication of digoxin toxicity. In this case, digoxin induces a variable degree of atrioventricular block as well as triggering the discharge of an atrial ectopic focus. The atrial rate is generally 150–200 bpm, and the degree of atrioventricular block may fluctuate producing an irregular ventricular rhythm. When atrial tachycardia with variable block complicates digoxin therapy:

1. Withhold further digoxin therapy until the arrhythmia resolves
2. Give beta-blockers (if necessary) to slow the ventricular rate
3. Ensure that potassium is above 4.0 mmol/l.

DC cardioversion should be avoided, as it may induce intractable arrhythmias in a patient with digoxin toxicity.

Multifocal atrial tachycardia most commonly arises as a complication of respiratory disease in acutely ill elderly patients, and is characterized by multiple atrial foci producing constant variation in the P-wave morphology and a variable atrial rate. Therapy consists of ensuring that the potassium level is adequate, and treating the underlying respiratory problem.

Ventricular tachyarrhythmias

In many patients with ischaemic heart disease, the first presentation is with a ventricular tachyarrhythmia leading to sudden cardiac death without any clear preceding history of MI or angina. Some patients present with a symptomatic sustained ventricular arrhythmia which may be related to underlying ischaemic heart disease or to other less common conditions, and this section deals with the investigation and treatment of these patients.

Ventricular tachycardia

Symptomatic sustained VT lasting for more than 30 seconds can occur without the occurrence of a recent MI. The most common cause is re-entry in scar tissue associated with an old MI. VT occurs less commonly in association with ventricular scarring in patients with previous cardiac surgery, with electrolyte abnormalities (hypokalaemia, hyperkalaemia and hypomagnesaemia) in patients with a long QT interval (which may be congenital or induced by drugs such as antiarrhythmic agents, antihistamines, tricyclic antidepressants, phenothiazines or erythro-mycin), in association with right ventricular disease, and (occasionally) in patients with structurally normal hearts.

Patients with VT present with symptoms associated with a broad complex tachycardia. A broad complex tachycardia can also be supra-ventricular in origin in patients with pre-existing or rate related bundle branch block or an accessory pathway. The important points to remember in a patient with a broad complex tachycardia are that:

1. VT is a common cause of broad complex tachycardia. Supraventricular arrhythmias are uncommon as a cause of broad complex tachycardia. *If you are in doubt about the diagnosis, treat the arrhythmia as VT.*

2. If there is a past medical history of ischaemic heart disease or cardiomyo-pathy, always treat a broad complex tachycardia as VT.

3. *Never give IV verapamil to a patient with a broad complex tachycardia, as it may cause severe and intractable haemodynamic depression if the tachycardia is VT.*

4. The patient's general clinical state is no guide to the site of origin of the tachycardia. The degree of haemodynamic compromise that occurs depends on the tachycardia rate and the patient's left ventricular function. Thus a rapid tachycardia of supraventricular origin may cause haemodynamic collapse in a patient with pre-existing left ventricular dysfunction or valvular heart disease, while a slow monomorphic VT may

be well tolerated in a patient with previous MI but relatively well preserved left ventricular function.

5. If the rhythm is irregular, the underlying tachycardia is commonly AF with bundle branch block. Less commonly, an irregular broad complex tachycardia with variable QRS morphology will be due to AF in a patient with an accessory pathway.

6. In patients who are not severely haemodynamically compromised, clinical assessment and the 12 lead ECG may aid in identifying the site of origin of a broad complex tachycardia (Figure 18.5, Table 18.1). Detailed analysis of the QRS morphology may further aid the diagnosis, but the criteria are complex to apply.

7. Adenosine can be used as a diagnostic aid in a patient with haemodynamically tolerated broad complex tachycardia. Since it has a very short half-life, it is well tolerated and safe to use in VT. If the arrhythmia is terminated by adenosine, it is almost certainly an AVNRT or AVRT. If the arrhythmia is unaffected by adenosine, it is almost certainly VT. Transient atrioventricular nodal blockade will reveal the underlying atrial activity in AF, atrial flutter or atrial tachycardia.

The immediate management of a patient with broad complex tachycardia is therefore as follows:

1. In a patient with severe haemodynamic compromise, immediate DC cardioversion with CPR (if necessary) is the treatment of choice.

2. If the tachycardia is haemodynamically tolerated (systolic BP >90 mmHg, conscious level normal, no chest pain or heart failure), carry out a clinical assessment and obtain a 12 lead ECG. Administer adenosine if there is any remaining diagnostic uncertainty. If VT is likely, treat as detailed in Chapter 8. If a supraventricular origin is likely, treat as detailed earlier in this chapter.

Following an episode of VT, careful evaluation by an electrophysiologist is necessary. Exercise testing or coronary angiography may be necessary, as reversible ischaemia associated with coronary artery disease is a common cause of VT. In younger patients, particularly if the VT is provoked by exercise, if there is a left bundle branch block morphology to the tachycardia or if there are T-wave or ST changes in V1 to V3, the VT may be related to right ventricular disease and MRI scanning will be necessary. Drug pro-arrhythmia, metabolic disturbance and congenital long QT syndromes need to be excluded.

If no readily reversible precipitating factor can be identified, electrophysiological testing may induce the arrhythmia and identify a drug capable of suppressing its induction. If a successful drug cannot be identified by electrophysiological testing, implantation of an AICD will

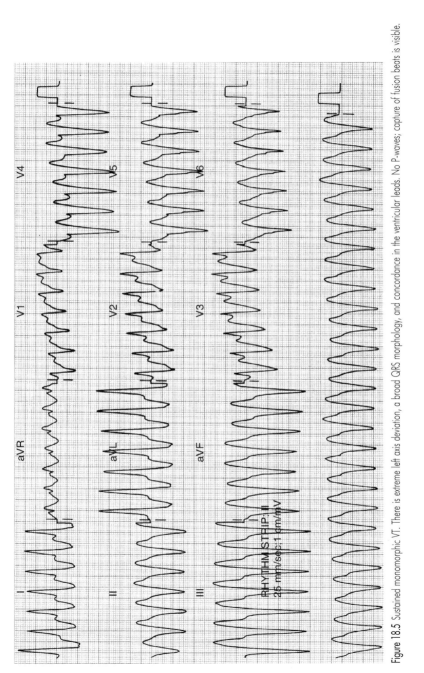

Figure 18.5 Sustained monomorphic VT. There is extreme left axis deviation, a broad QRS morphology, and concordance in the ventricular leads. No P-waves; capture of fusion beats is visible.

Table 18.1 Identification of site of origin of broad complex tachycardia based on clinical or electrocardiographic features.

Ventricular origin	Supraventricular origin
Clinical evidence of AV dissociation present (Cannon waves or variable intensity S1)	Clinical evidence of AV dissociation absent
ECG evidence of AV dissociation present (independent P-wave activity, fusion beats or capture beats)	ECG evidence of AV dissociation absent
QRS width >140 ms	QRS width <140 ms
Concordant activation pattern in ventricular leads	Discordant activation pattern in ventricular leads
Deep S-wave in V6 present	Deep S-wave in V6 absent
RSr pattern in V1 (with primary R-wave taller than secondary R-wave)	RSr pattern in V1 absent

improve prognosis. If invasive assessment is inappropriate, empirical therapy with amiodarone is better than other agents.

Torsade de pointes ventricular tachycardia

Torsade de pointes ventricular tachycardia is polymorphic VT that occurs in association with QT prolongation. The arrhythmia commonly occurs as a complication of Class I or Class III antiarrhythmic drug therapy. Other less common causes are:

1. Other drugs such as tricyclic antidepressants, phenothiazines, some antihistamines and erythromycin
2. Electrolyte abnormalities (hypokalaemia, hypomagnesaemia)
3. Congenital abnormalities of cardiac repolarization
4. Profound bradycardia.

Torsade presents as non-sustained and repetitive episodes of polymorphic VT, which appears to rotate around the isoelectric line (Figure 18.6). Treatment is as follows:

1. DC cardioversion plus cardiopulmonary resuscitation (if necessary) for any prolonged episodes associated with cardiorespiratory arrest
2. Withdrawal of precipitating drugs
3. Intravenous magnesium using the regime detailed in Chapter 24

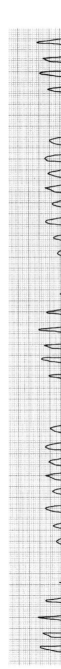

Figure 18.6 Torsades de Pointes. Rapid, polymorphic VT that appears to rotate around the isoelectric line.

4. Correction of hypokalaemia (if present) using the regime detailed in Chapter 24.

If the above treatment fails to prevent episodes of torsade de pointes, temporary ventricular pacing at a rate of 100 bpm will shorten the QT interval and may be effective. If further episodes occur, increasing the pacing rate may be beneficial. In patients with congenital long QT syndrome, attacks of torsade de pointes usually occur in association with increased sympathetic tone, and therapy with beta-blockers, surgical sympathectomy or a pacing system may be indicated after careful evaluation by an electrophysiologist.

Bradyarrhythmias

Symptomatic bradyarrhythmias are not always associated with acute MI. Age-related degenerative disease of the conduction system or atrioventricular nodal blocking drugs often produce symptoms of dizziness or syncope associated with intermittent or permanent bradycardia. Examination of the 12 lead ECG usually shows evidence of conduction system disease with bifasicular or trifasicular block, established atrioventricular block, or evidence of sick sinus syndrome. In a patient with a history of dizziness or syncope and electrocardiographic evidence of conduction system disease:

1. If profound bradycardia is present, an isoprenaline infusion (see Chapter 24) or external cardiac pacing will provide rhythm support until a temporary pacing wire can be positioned.

2. If complete heart block with a slow (<40 bpm) or broad complex rhythm is present, episodes of ventricular standstill may occur unpredictably, as the subsidiary pacemaker responsible for the escape rhythm is often unreliable. A temporary pacemaker should be inserted. Manipulation of temporary pacing leads within the heart often precipitates ventricular standstill in these patients. If possible, an isoprenaline infusion (see Chapter 24) should be readily available before the procedure is commenced.

3. If complete heart block with a faster (>40 bpm) narrow complex rhythm is present, it is reasonable to initially observe the patient on CCU. The risks associated with temporary pacemaker insertion (particularly by an inexperienced operator) probably exceed the risk associated with an initial policy of observation, since this type of escape rhythm is usually reliable and the risk of sudden prolonged ventricular standstill is low. If prolonged pauses do occur, proceed to temporary pacing.

4. If the initial rhythm is sinus with an adequate rate but there is a suspicion

Key points

- Most tachyarrhythmias can be treated using only three antiarrhythmic agents (adenosine, lignocaine and amiodarone).

- AF is a common cause of exercise capacity limitation, and is associated with a significant risk of thromboembolism. Most patients with recent onset AF should receive treatment aimed at restoring sinus rhythm (usually with intravenous amiodarone).

- Atrial flutter is less common than AF, and is often resistant to drug therapy.

- The commonest cause of paroxysmal narrow complex tachycardia is AVNRT, which usually responds to intravenous adenosine.

- Accessory pathways (which may be concealed) are a common cause of paroxysmal narrow complex tachycardia. The ECG often shows a narrow complex tachycardia, with P-waves visible between complexes. AF may be dangerous, and all patients suspected of having an accessory pathway should be assessed by an electrophysiologist.

- Unifocal atrial tachycardia is rare, and is often resistant to drug therapy. Atrial tachycardia with block may arise as a complication of digoxin toxicity, and polymorphic atrial tachycardia as a complication of respiratory disease.

- Broad complex tachycardia may be supraventricular in origin, but VT is a more common cause. If in any doubt, treat as VT. *Never use IV verapamil in a patient with broad complex tachycardia.*

- The appropriate treatment for torsade de pointes is magnesium or pacing, and not antiarrhythmic drugs.

- Many bradyarrhythmias can be treated with initial observation. Temporary pacing is required for complete heart block with a slow or broad complex escape rhythm.

of intermittent conduction block or bradyarrhythmia, admit to CCU for rhythm monitoring.

Following admission, drugs that may be responsible for the bradyarrhythmia should be withdrawn and other treatable abnormalities such as thyroid dysfunction or MI excluded. If there is no easily reversible cause for the bradyarrhythmia, implantation of a permanent pacing system may be indicated.

References

Channer, K. S. (1996). Treatment of atrial fibrillation. *Prescribers Journal*, **36**, 146–153.

Cobbe, S. M. (1997). Using the right drug: a treatment algorithm for atrial fibrillation. *Eur. Heart J.*, **18**, C33–C39.

Dancy, M. and Ward, D. (1989). Diagnosis of ventricular tachycardia: a clinical algorithm. *Br. Med. J.*, **291**, 1036–1038.

Fresco, C. and Proclemer, A. (1996). Management of recent onset atrial fibrillation. *Eur. Heart J.*, **17** (Suppl. C), 41–47.

Ganz, L. J. and Friedman, P. L. (1995). Supraventricular tachycardia. *N. Engl. J. Med.*, **332**, 162–173.

Levy, S. and Ricard, P. (1997). Using the right drup: a treatment algorithm for regular supraventriculat tachycardias. *Eur. Heart J.*, **18**, C27–C32.

Lip, G. Y. H., Watson, R. D. S. and Singh, S. P. (1996). Cardioversion of atrial fibrillation. *Br. Med. J.*, **312**, 112–115.

Obel, O. A. and Camm, A. J. (1997). Supraventricular tachycardia. ECG diagnosis and anatomy. *Eur. Heart J.*, **18**, C2–C11.

Pye, M., Camm, A. J. (1996). Supraventricular tachycardia. *Hospital Update*, **22**, 226–237.

Rankin, A. C. and Cobbe, S. M. (1993). Broad complex tachycardias. *Prescribers Journal*, **33**, 138–146.

Ruden, D. M. (1994). Risks and benefits of antiarrhythmic therapy. *N. Engl. J. Med.*, **331**, 785–791.

Sopher, S. M. and Camun, A. J. (1996). Atrial fibrillation: Maintenance of sinus rhythm versus rate control. *Am. J. Cardiol.*, **77**, 24A–37A.

Winner, S. and Boon, N. (1979). Clinical problems with temporary pacemakers prior to permanent pacing. *J. R. Coll. Physicians Lond.*, **23**, 161–163.

19

Emergency treatment of hypertension

Background

Severe uncontrolled hypertension is now uncommon in developed countries, as a result of better control of blood pressure generally. Poorly controlled severe hypertension in the absence of life-threatening complications is usually treated with standard oral antihypertensive agents. In these patients, blood pressure should be reduced over a period of two to three days, thereby avoiding ischaemic renal and neurological damage. In hypertensive emergencies (Table 19.1), sustained severe hypertension is associated with life-threatening renal, cardiovascular or neurological complications. Rapid control of blood pressure is required (usually with a parenteral agent) to avoid the associated high levels of morbidity and mortality. One should be aware that too rapid a reduction in BP may have adverse renal and neurological effects, and therefore controlled reduction of BP over the course of a few hours should be achieved with the target diastolic BP in the region of 100–110 mmHg. After a period of stability at the target BP lasting 6–48 hours, oral therapy can be commenced and the parenteral agents 'tailed off'.

Table 19.1 Hypertensive emergencies

Hypertensive LVF
Hypertensive encephalopathy
Hypertension with unstable angina or MI
Hypertension with aortic dissection
Phaeochromocytoma crisis
Eclampsia or severe pre-eclampsia
Hypertension with acute renal failure
Severe hypertension with interocerebral haemorrhage or acute subarachnoid haemorrhage

Table 19.2 Drugs used for the treatment of hypertensive crisis.

Nitroprusside	Rapid onset and short duration of action Useful in heart failure, encephalopathy, aortic dissection
Nitroglycerine	Rapid onset and short duration of action Useful in heart failure and MI
Atenolol	5 mg boluses, titrated against BP and heart rate. Useful in the presence of myocardial ischaemia/infarction and aortic dissection
Labetalol	Onset 5–10 minutes, duration 1–8 hours. Given as bolus or infusion in eclampsia
Hydralazine	Onset 10–20 minutes, duration 4–6 hours. Often used in eclampsia. Given as bolus or infusion

The use of sublingual antihypertensive agents (e.g. nifedipine) should generally be avoided due to the unpredictable and uncontrolled BP lowering, which is not readily reversible. This has been associated with increased mortality from cerebrovascular events, so at best this should be restricted only to situations where the facilities for parenteral medication are not readily available.

Table 19.2 lists a variety of parenteral antihypertensive agents available for the treatment of hypertensive emergencies. Some specific management strategies follow.

Hypertensive emergencies

Malignant hypertension

Malignant hypertension is diagnosed by the findings of severe hypertension (diastolic BP usually >130 mmHg) together with bilateral retinal haemorrhages and exudates, with or without papilloedema. It is more common in middle age, in ethnic subgroups such as Afro-Caribbeans and in smokers, with a worse prognosis in the presence of renal failure. There is no indication for the use of parenteral therapy in the absence of other complications, such as LVF or encephalopathy. Beta-blockers (e.g. atenolol) and calcium antagonists (e.g. nifedipine) are useful first line agents. Combination therapy with diuretics, ACE inhibitors or other vasodilators may be required for long-term control.

Hypertensive left ventricular failure (LVF)

Hypertensive LVF is a heterogeneous disorder with severity ranging from acute fulminating pulmonary oedema to a more chronic form of heart failure. This has led to the recommendation that morphine, oxygen and frusemide IV should be given to all patients, with IV sodium nitroprusside or nitroglycerine (especially in patients with myocardial ischaemia) for acute pulmonary oedema.

When heart failure and renal failure co-exist in patients who are severely hypertensive, bilateral renal artery stenosis should be suspected. Moreover, although ACE inhibitors have a survival advantage in heart failure, the risk of precipitating renal failure in patients with undiagnosed bilateral renal artery stenosis means that the safest strategy is probably to avoid an ACE inhibitor until renovascular disease can be excluded.

Where patients have previously been treated with agents with a negatively inotropic action such as beta-blockers or verapamil, these should be discontinued.

Hypertensive encephalopathy

Hypertensive encephalopathy is a heterogeneous condition whose clinical presentation may vary, thus making management difficult. It results from a breakdown in cerebral autoregulation and is characterized by altered consciousness, ranging from confusion to coma, seizures, transient hemiparesis, visual loss and other focal signs. Severe headache, nausea, vomiting and advanced fundal changes are the most common features.

When hypertensive encephalopathy has developed on a background of chronic hypertension, there may be a greater risk of ischaemic complications associated with rapid blood pressure reduction than when encephalopathy has arisen *de novo*. It is therefore inadvisable to lower diastolic BP below 100 mmHg. When symptoms have been present for days or weeks, oral treatment is, therefore, probably safest. When, however, it is felt that irreversible neurological damage will occur within hours, IV control of BP is necessary. Ideally this should be with sodium nitroprusside, as it has a rapid onset and short duration of activity, making it easy to titrate against the BP and to avoid precipitous falls in pressure. The main side-effect, however, is thiocyanate toxicity, which limits the prolonged use of the drug and also its use in renal failure.

Hypertension with unstable angina or MI

The hypertension in acute coronary conditions is usually transient, due to pain and catecholamine release. The hypertensive response can increase myocardial oxygen demand and potentiate myocardial ischaemia and necrosis. Hypertension in the early stages of MI increases the risk of intracranial haemorrhage when thrombolytic therapy is used, and has an adverse effect on long-term survival. Many patients will revert to a normotensive state after relief of pain and anxiety. When the hypertension persists, a more detailed assessment is required, including obtaining a history of prior hypertension, previous treatment and whether such therapy has recently been withdrawn. With sustained hypertension in the absence of heart failure and heart block, beta-blockers should be considered the first line therapy due to their prognostic benefit. These can be used IV in conjunction with the administration of thrombolysis. Second line therapy should be IV nitrates, as these have a neutral effect on long-term prognosis.

Hypertension with aortic dissection

See Chapter 20.

Phaeochromocytoma crises

Phaeochromocytomas are tumours of the sympatho-adrenal system, arising from chromaffin cells. Most are intra-abdominal and benign, with about 10 per cent being familial. They can all secrete many different catecholamines, but mainly noradrenaline is produced. Symptoms of catecholamine excess include headache, sweating, palpitations/tachycardia, tremor, nausea/vomiting, anxiety, and chest or abdominal pain. Attacks are abrupt and of variable duration due to the intermittent nature of catecholamine secretion. The blood pressure is characteristically labile. Acute hypertensive crises require control with IV alpha antagonists such as phentolamine (3–5 mg). Beta-blockers should not be given before alpha-blockade, as this will exacerbate the hypertension due to unopposed alpha vasoconstrictor activity. However, after the administration of an alpha-blocker, beta-blockers are useful for the treatment of tachycardias and arrhythmias. In addition, there should be intra-arterial BP monitoring and plasma volume expansion as patients are often hypovolaemic.

Eclampsia or severe pre-eclampsia

Pre-eclampsia (proteinuria and a rise in BP to over 140/90 mmHg during the second half of pregnancy) and eclampsia (with additional oedema, central nervous system signs, convulsions, renal failure, pulmonary oedema and/or disseminated intravascular coagulation) remain common causes of both maternal and foetal mortality. The management of these conditions is complex, and should be undertaken by a senior obstetrician. Generally, depending on the severity of the condition, oral labetalol or nifedipine have proven value and safety. Hydralazine can also be used in the emergency situation; however, ACE inhibitors and thiazide diuretics should be avoided. Once blood pressure has been controlled, a management plan is instigated by a senior obstetrician with a decision on the use of anticonvulsants and the timing of delivery.

Key points

- In the absence of life-threatening complications, elevated BP should be lowered gradually with oral medication, to avoid ischaemic end organ damage.

- The sublingual route of administration for therapy (e.g. nifedipine) should be avoided.

- Parenteral therapy should be reserved for emergency situations which are life-threatening or associated with major complications.

References

Calhoun, D. A. and Oparil, S. (1990). Treatment of hypertensive crises. *N. Engl. J. Med.*, **323**, 1177–1183.

Grossman, E., Messerli, F. H., Grodzicki, T., *et al.* (1996). Should a moratorium be placed on sublingual nifedipine capsules given for hypertensive emergencies and pseudo emergencies? *JAMA*, **276**(16), 1328–1331.

Kaplan, N. M. (1994). Management of hypertensive emergencies. *Lancet*, **344**, 1335–1338.

20

Acute aortic disease

Aortic dissection

Background

Acute aortic dissection is an uncommon yet potentially catastrophic clinical event. The incidence is approximately five to ten per million population per year. Males are affected at least twice as often as females, and it is more common in Africans than Caucasians. The usual age range is 50–70 years; however, it is not an uncommon cause of sudden death in younger subjects. Untreated, the condition carries a mortality of one to three per cent per hour over the first 48 hours. Centres with an active interest in the evaluation and management of acute dissection have lowered hospital mortality rates to 15–25 per cent. Diagnosis begins with a high degree of clinical suspicion, when a patient presents with chest pain and one or more predisposing risk factors (see below), most notably hypertension or an inherited disorder of connective tissue.

Risk factors

1. Hypertension (major risk factor in more than 50 per cent of patients)

2. Bicuspid aortic valve

3. Coarctation of the aorta

4. Pregnancy

5. Turner's or Noonan's syndrome

6. Marfan's syndrome

7. Vasculitic disorders e.g., SLE, Ehlers Danlos

8. Surgical aortotomy sites.

Pathophysiology

The dissection is usually spontaneous, and occurs following the sudden development of an intimal tear in the aorta. A combination of high luminal pressure and/or medial disease (due to elastic fibre or smooth muscle cell degeneration) are the rule. The majority ($\sim$70 per cent) of acute dissections arise in the ascending aorta, 1–3 cm distal to the coronary ostia (this being the area subject to maximum haemodynamic and torsional stress). The second most frequent site of entry is distal to the left subclavian artery, where the relatively mobile arch becomes anchored to the thoracic wall by the ligamentum arteriosum. As the tear develops, blood at systemic pressure is driven into the aortic wall, splitting it along the plane of least resistance and so producing the acute dissection. The dissection propagates for varying distances throughout the aorta, usually in an antegrade direction, although retrograde spread can and does occur. Alternatively, the dissecting haematoma can rupture through the adventitia into the pleural or pericardial cavity, and will lead to rapid death in the majority of patients before they reach hospital.

An important pathological variant of aortic dissection is intramural haemorrhage (IMH) without an intimal flap, which may occur in as many as 20 per cent of patients with suspected dissection. Patients with IMH cannot be distinguished from classic dissection on clinical grounds, and they show the same potential for aortic regurgitation, pulse deficits and neurological syndromes. The frequent progression of IMH to either dissection or rupture has led to the suggestion that the management strategy should be the same as that for classic dissection.

Classification

Many classification systems have been proposed, based on the location and extent of dissection. The relevance of these is that patients with proximal dissection are at high risk of aortic root and cerebrovascular complications, and surgical management has been demonstrated to be superior. Patients with distal dissection are at lower risk, and are best managed medically. The Stanford classification system is most widely used, and divides dissections into type A or type B.

Type A is any dissection involving the ascending aorta, regardless of site of intimal tear.

Type B is when the dissection process is restricted to the aorta distal to the left subclavian artery.

Clinical features

1. Presence of a risk factor (hypertension or connective tissue disorder).
2. Pain: typically severe and of sudden onset; described as a tearing pain, often located in the intrascapular area and possibly radiating to the neck or arms, or retrosternally. The pain may be similar to ischaemic pain, and dissection around a coronary artery ostium may produce an additional MI. Leaking aneurysms may cause pleuritic chest pain.
3. Symptoms/signs from arterial involvement may include:
   a. monoplegia, paraplegia (due to spinal artery involvement)
   b. hemiplegia (due to dissection of head and neck vessels)
   c. loss of consciousness
   d. abdominal pain (mesenteric artery)
   e. dysphagia (oesophageal compression)
   f. pain and pallor in limb or limbs
   g. pulse deficits.
4. Shortness of breath, which may be due to LVF, haemothorax or pleural/pericardial effusions.
5. The blood pressure may be elevated, normal or low. BP in both arms should be documented; there may be a discrepancy, depending on the site of dissection.
6. Presence of new aortic regurgitation.

Diagnosis

NB: *A high index of clinical suspicion is of key importance!*

A CXR classically shows a widened upper mediastinum and may also demonstrate fluid in the left costophrenic angle. There may be separation of the line of aortic calcification >0.5 cm from the outline of the aorta at the aortic arch.

An ECG may be normal, or show evidence of LVH, ischaemia or acute infarction.

If aortic dissection is suspected, contact a senior colleague immediately. Emergency treatment is as follows:

1. Control pain with intravenous diamorphine.
2. Reduce and control BP (to minimize aortic wall shear stress and limit further extension), aiming for a peak systolic pressure of 100–120 mmHg using IV beta-blockade (labetalol, atenolol).
3. If the blood pressure cannot be adequately controlled with beta-blockade, then an infusion of nitroprusside or nitroglycerine can be added as second line treatment. These should not be used without prior

beta-blockade, as nitrate induced vasodilatation may cause an increase in the rate of rise of arterial pressure and so increase shear stress in the aortic wall.

4. Ensure good venous access and group and cross-match blood.

Subsequent investigations to confirm the diagnosis will depend on local availability and expertise, as imaging techniques are rapidly evolving. These may include:

1. Contrast aortography. Previous gold standard technique; however, there may be delays in access to a vascular lab and the procedure carries a recognized risk. It may also be the least sensitive technique for detecting IMH.

2. Transthoracic echo, to look for the size of the aortic root, aortic regurgitation and pericardial fluid. Occasionally a flap can be seen. Views of aortic arch and descending aorta are limited.

3. Transoesophageal echocardiography (TOE) with analgesia and sedation. This investigation has a high sensitivity and specificity, and will frequently determine the extent of the dissection and differentiate the true from the false lumen. In addition, it can be performed on the coronary/ intensive care unit, where monitoring and management can continue uninterrupted.

4. MRI or contrast-enhanced CT scanning can both give excellent diagnostic accuracy; however, the patient has to be moved to the radiology department. These are the investigations of choice where TOE is not possible or not diagnostic.

Management

In addition to the above measures, proximal (type A) dissections require immediate surgical repair to prevent the complications of tamponade, coronary dissection, aortic rupture or stroke. The ascending aorta is excised and if the valve is involved the cusps are resuspended. If this is not possible, the valve is replaced. Distal dissections are treated medically unless there is evidence of end-organ malperfusion or threat to a limb.

Follow up and prognosis

Early surgical repair has transformed the prognosis of type A lesions, with survival in excess of 80 per cent. Aggressive medical therapy for type B lesions results in ~85 per cent early survival. All patients with dissection require careful follow up, meticulous BP control and regular screening to detect redissection or aneurysm formation, particularly in patients with Marfan's syndrome.

Traumatic rupture of the aorta

Background

Aortic rupture is a relatively common injury, and estimates suggest it causes death in 10–15 per cent of road traffic accidents. Most of these will occur at the trauma scene as the result of sudden, massive exsanguination. In general, the majority of victims are aged under 45, with men affected twice as often as women.

Mechanism

The commonest cause is from blunt chest trauma due to a motor vehicle accident. As a result of rapid deceleration of the thorax and compression of the diaphragm, the aorta is subjected to extreme torque and compression. This is maximal at its points of attachment, the sinuses of Valsalva, the isthmus (just distal to the origin of the left subclavian artery) and the diaphragm.

It is postulated that the relatively mobile heart and great vessels continue to move forward while the descending aorta does not, being 'fixed' to the vertebral column by the intercostal arteries and surrounding fascia. The severe aortic wall stress results in rupture through the intima, often continuing into the media and adventitia. The extent of the forces involved will dictate the degree of aortic transection. Transection is frequently complete, but with lesser violence, parts of the aortic wall may remain intact in the presence of a tear in a portion of its circumference (usually posteriorly).

Approximately 70 per cent of acute aortic transections occur in the upper descending thoracic aorta, as a result of horizontal deceleration forces. In accidents with vertical deceleration (e.g. falls from a great height and aircraft accidents), the tear is commonly in the ascending aorta or arch. Blast injuries, crush injuries and other direct trauma may also cause rupture. In many of these cases there is more than one tear.

Clinical features

The presence of severe injuries to the limbs, head, abdomen and central nervous system often masks the diagnosis of aortic injury. There is always a history of abrupt deceleration or direct trauma, but only two-thirds of patients have external evidence of thoracic trauma (contusion, rib or vertebral fractures and haemorrhagic pleural effusions). Therefore, a high index of suspicion is necessary in order to make a prompt diagnosis.

Patients who survive to reach the hospital may have profound haemor-rhagic shock; some, however, are haemodynamically stable after initial resuscitative measures. In a small number of cases there is paradoxical upper limb hypertension with hypotension in the legs, and a posteriorly heard systolic murmur. Evidence of impaired blood flow distal to the transection is uncommon; a minority of patients may have lower limb ischaemia or paraplegia. Few symptoms are directly attributable to the aortic trauma itself. Stable, conscious patients may experience pain radiating to the back, as in aortic dissection. Pressure from a localized expanding haematoma can cause dyspnoea and stridor (due to tracheal or bronchial constriction), dysphagia (oesophageal compression) or SVC obstruction.

Diagnosis

The diagnosis must be suspected in any patient with severe injuries. In the absence of classical physical findings (which is common), the diagnosis is best suspected from the CXR, which is usually abnormal, although the abnormalities are variable. No finding on the CXR is diagnostic, but possible abnormalities include:

1. Widened mediastinum
2. Tracheal or nasogastric tube deviation to the right
3. Blurring of the usually well defined aortic outline
4. Downward displacement of the left main bronchus
5. Left haemothorax
6. Opacification of the subaortic window.

TOE is an effective means of imaging the aortic arch and descending aorta. A recent study suggests that TOE may compare favourably with arch aortography, being highly sensitive and specific, but clinical ex-pertise is limited. In addition, TOE can be performed safely and quickly, at the same time as other procedures and at the bedside, so the critically injured patient does not have to be moved. However in patients with multiple trauma it does require considerable skill, and it should be avoided in patients with unstable spinal injuries. An equivocal or negative TOE result should be followed by aortography. Aortography (carried out via the arm) was the gold standard investigation, although fatal complications have been reported. The typical diagnostic features are of a pseudoaneurysm at the isthmus, and a visible tear or leak. CT and MRI scanning are less satisfactory than aortography or TOE. Scanning is often used to exclude haematoma in patients with an abnormal mediastinal outline who are undergoing scans for other reasons relating to their traumatic injury.

Management and prognosis

The prognosis of aortic transection is very poor. Only 15 per cent of patients reach hospital alive, and 50 per cent of these will die within 48 hours without surgery. Once a tear has been identified, early operation is indicated. If surgery has to be delayed while other injuries are dealt with, medical management is with beta-blockade to strictly control blood pressure and cardiac contractility. In general, 75–85 per cent of patients undergoing surgery can be expected to leave hospital.

Penetrating ulcers of the aorta

Background

This condition tends to have the same clinical presentation as aortic dissection, and should therefore be considered in the differential diagnosis of acute chest/back pain. However, the pathophysiology is different, with these ulcers tending to complicate aortic atherosclerosis. Their development is thought to be as a result of an atherosclerotic plaque eroding and ulcerating through the internal elastic lamina and into the media. This produces a variable amount of intramural haematoma, although it tends not to be associated with extensive longitudinal propagation, due to the coexisting fibrosis that occurs with long-standing atherosclerosis. This process may be further complicated by pseudo-aneurysm formation, aneurysmal dilatation or aortic rupture. The ulcers may be single or multiple, and can involve the entire aorta, although they tend to occur most commonly in the mid to distal descending thoracic aorta.

Clinical features

Patients tend to be elderly, with multiple risk factors for atherosclerotic disease. Most present with symptoms of chest or back pain; however, they tend not have the associated valvular, pericardial or neurovascular complications seen with classic dissection and IMH. In addition, they may present with symptoms of distal ischaemia caused by emboli arising from the ulcerated atheroma.

Diagnosis

As discussed above, the diagnosis of acute aortic syndromes has been greatly enhanced by improved imaging techniques, including angiography, CT, MRI and TOE. The particular diagnostic strategy adopted by any institution will depend on local availability and expertise.

Management

Treatment for acute aortic ulceration remains controversial, particularly with respect to the indications for surgical resection. Many patients have been successfully managed conservatively with medical therapy, which includes control of blood pressure and serial follow up with imaging tests to detect complications. Indications for surgery include haemorrhage, recurrent chest/back pain, embolization, enlarging pseudoaneurysm and aneurysmal dilatation. Until the natural history of this condition is defined, it will remain unknown on presentation which patients can be managed adequately with non-operative therapy.

Key points

- Spontaneous aortic dissection occurs most commonly in hypertensive males aged 50–70 years, and has a high mortality.

- Most dissections arise in the ascending aorta, and these require surgical repair.

- There is a high index of suspicion for a dissection in a patient with severe chest pain and a normal ECG.

- Remember that the absence of pulse deficits, or a normal CXR, do not exclude a dissection.

- If a dissection tracks down into the aortic root, it may involve the origin of the coronary arteries (particularly the right) and produce ECG and clinical signs of an MI in addition to the dissection.

- TOE or CT/MRI can be used to diagnose aortic dissection, if available.

- Traumatic rupture of the aorta should be suspected in all cases of RTA or falls from a height. This is a lethal condition, and requires urgent investigation by a senior cardiologist with a view to immediate surgical repair if possible.

References

Braverman, A. C. (1994). Penetrating atherosclerotic ulcers of the aorta. *Curr. Opin. Cardiol.*, **9**, 591–597.

Dapunt, O. E., Galla, J. D., Sadegift, A. M., *et al.* (1994). The natural history of thoracic aortic aneurysms. *J. Thoracic Cardiovasc. Surg.*, **107**, 1323–1333.

Nienaber, C. A., Spielmann, R. P., Von Kodolitsch, Y., *et al.* (1992). Diagnosis of thoracic aortic dissection: magnetic resonance imaging versus transesophageal echocardiography. *Circulation*, **85**, 433–437.

O'Gara, P. T., Roman, W. and DeSanctis, W. (1995). Acute aortic dissection and its variants. Toward a common diagnostic and therapeutic approach. *Circulation*, **92**, 1376–1378.

Smith, M. D., Cassidy, J. M., Souther, S., *et al.* (1995). Transesophageal echocardiography in the diagnosis of traumatic rupture of the aorta. *N. Engl. J. Med.*, **332**, 356–362.

Wheat, M. W. (1980). Acute dissecting aneurysms of the aorta: diagnosis and treatment – 1979. *Am. Heart J.*, **99**, 373–387.

21

Pulmonary embolism

Background

Pulmonary embolism is a common problem in hospitalized patients, contributing to 10–20 per cent of all deaths. The majority (>90 per cent) of all PEs originate from deep venous thrombosis in the leg veins. Untreated PE has a 30 per cent mortality, but anticoagulation provides immediate and almost complete protection against recurrent embolism and reduces the death rate to less than 10 per cent. Mortality from PE is highest in patients with pre-existing cardiorespiratory disease. It is more difficult to interpret the results of V/Q scans in these patients, and spiral CT or pulmonary angiography may be necessary to clarify the diagnosis and guide therapy.

A variety of different conditions increase the risk of PE (Table 21.1). Deep venous thrombosis is common following acute MI, particularly in patients who have a complicated clinical course associated with heart failure, or prolonged bed rest. Post-infarction patients who have a complicated clinical course should be considered for prophylactic low dose subcutaneous heparin 5000 units bd. Despite the common occurrence of asymptomatic deep venous thrombosis, the incidence of fatal PE is less than one per cent in post-infarction patients.

The majority of patients with PE present with an acute minor embolism that obstructs less than 50 per cent of the pulmonary circulation and can be treated with anticoagulants and other supportive therapy. In 10 per cent of patients, an acute massive embolus obstructs more than 50 per cent of the pulmonary circulation and causes profound haemodynamic compromise. Mortality is high in patients with acute massive emboli, and invasive treatment designed to disrupt or lyse the emboli should be considered. The absence of clinical signs in the leg does not rule out a diagnosis of PE, as many deep venous thromboses are clinically silent.

Table 21.1 Risk factors for pulmonary embolism.

Recent surgery (particularly orthopaedic procedures), trauma or burns
Malignancy
Immobility
MI
Pregnancy and oral contraceptive usage
Increasing age
Heart failure
Inflammatory bowel disease
Coagulation disorders
Nephrotic syndrome

Acute massive PE

Patients who sustain an acute massive PE present with a combination of the following features:

1. Acute onset severe dyspnoea, wheeze and central cyanosis
2. Retrosternal chest pain
3. Syncope or collapse
4. Signs of major haemodynamic compromise (tachycardia, hypotension, raised jugular venous pressure and low cardiac output)
5. Abnormal electrocardiogram with sinus tachycardia, AF, $S_IQ_{III}T_{III}$ pattern, signs of right heart strain
6. Oligaemic segments on CXR
7. Severe hypoxia, acidosis and low PCO_2 due to impaired gas exchange and tachypnoea
8. Echocardiographic right ventricular dilatation and abnormal septal motion.

If the diagnosis of acute massive PE cannot confidently be made on the basis of clinical features, electrocardiogram, blood gases, CXR and transthoracic echocardiography, urgent spiral CT or pulmonary angiography are indicated to guide appropriate therapy.

Treatment of acute massive PE is as follows:

1. Administer high concentration oxygen to improve gas exchange, and intravenous diamorphine to reduce distress.
2. Commence intravenous heparin with a 5000 unit bolus followed by an infusion of 20 000 units 12 hourly (with the infusion rate titrated to maintain APTT 2–3 times control).
3. Consult a senior colleague regarding thrombolytic therapy. If there are

no contraindications, lytic therapy will speed the resolution of clots and improve haemodynamics. The fastest acting agent is rt-PA, which should be administered using the regime detailed in Chapter 24.

4. If life-threatening haemodynamic compromise is present, consult a senior colleague regarding emergency pulmonary angiography. Major clots can be mechanically disrupted with specialized catheters. In certain circumstances, emergency surgical pulmonary embolectomy may be considered.

Acute minor PE

Patients who sustain an acute minor PE do not have major haemodynamic compromise. Blood pressure is usually normal, and the venous pressure is not raised. Patients with acute minor PE present with a combination of the following features:

1. Dyspnoea, pleuritic chest pain or haemoptysis

2. Moderate hypoxia, fever or tachycardia

3. Abnormal electrocardiogram with sinus tachycardia, AF or ST/T wave changes in V1–V3

4. Pulmonary shadowing, a raised hemidiaphragm or pleural effusion on CXR

5. No evidence of echocardiographic right ventricular abnormalities.

If a diagnosis of minor PE is suspected on clinical grounds, institute immediate intravenous anticoagulation with heparin. In the majority of patients the diagnosis can be confirmed by a combination of V/Q scanning and ultrasound examination of the leg veins, with spiral CT scanning or pulmonary angiography reserved for patients in whom clinical suspicion of PE remains high despite the results of V/Q and ultrasound. In the diagnosis of PE, the following guidelines are useful:

1. A high probability V/Q scan is associated with angiographically detectable PE in 97 per cent of cases, and anticoagulation is mandatory. No further diagnostic tests are necessary.

2. An intermediate scan or low probability scan is unreliable, and 40 per cent of these patients will have angiographically detectable PEs. These patients should have an ultrasound scan of the leg veins. If the leg ultrasound is positive, PE is likely and anticoagulation is indicated. If the ultrasound is negative and clinical probability is low, no further treatment or investigation is necessary. The risk of a further event in these patients is very low. If the leg ultrasound is negative but the clinical suspicion of PE is high, or the patient has pre-existing cardiorespiratory

disease, pulmonary angiography or spiral CT scanning is indicated to clarify the diagnosis and guide appropriate therapy.

3. A normal V/Q scan rules out a diagnosis of PE, and another cause of the patient's symptoms and signs should be sought.

If recurrent PE occurs despite adequate anticoagulant therapy, a vena-caval filter should be considered.

Key points

- PE is a common cause of death in hospitalized patients.

- Deep venous thrombosis (often clinically undetectable) is common following acute MI; fatal PE occurs in less than one per cent of patients.

- Acute massive PE is often associated with an abnormal ECG and transthoracic echocardiogram. Thrombolytic therapy or percutaneous thrombectomy may be life saving if haemodynamic compromise is severe.

- Acute minor PE is more difficult to diagnose. A high probability or normal V/Q scan provides clear evidence on which to base treatment. An intermediate or low probability scan is unreliable, and further investigation is indicated.

References

Davidson, B. L. and Deppert, E. J. (1998). Ultrasound for the diagnosis of deep vein thrombosis: where to now? *Br. Med. J.*, **316**, 2–3.

Fennerty, T. (1997). The diagnosis of pulmonary embolism. *Br. Med. J.*, **314**, 425–429.

Fennerty, T. (1998). Pulmonary embolism. *Br. Med. J.*, **317**, 91–92.

Goldhaber, S. Z. (1991). Thrombolysis for pulmonary embolism. *Prog. Cardiovasc. Dis.*, **34**, 113–134.

Hansell, D. and Flower, C. D. R. (1998). Imaging pulmonary embolism. A new look with spiral computed tomography. *Br. Med. J.*, **316**, 490–1.

Meneveau, N., Schiele, F., Vuillemenot, A. *et al.* (1997). Streptokinase vs. Altepase in massive pulmonary embolism. *Eur. Heart. J.*, **18**, 1141–1148.

Morrel, N. W. and Seed, W. A. (1992). Diagnosing pulmonary embolism. *Br. Med. J.*, **304**, 1126–1127.

Perrier, A. and Junod, A. F. (1995). Has the diagnosis of pulmonary embolism become easier to establish? *Resp. Med.*, **89**, 214–251.

22

Non-ischaemic cardiovascular emergencies

Pericarditis

Background

Pericarditis can result from any one of a number of inflammatory processes affecting the pericardium (Table 22.1). These may result in restriction of cardiac filling, either as a result of blood or fluid trapped in the pericardial sac (cardiac tamponade) or from thickening of the pericardium (constrictive pericarditis). Both conditions may be prevented if diagnosis and management are undertaken early.

Presentation

Pericarditis classically presents with chest pain, which is localized sub/retrosternally and exacerbated by breathing, coughing, moving or lying supine. Relief from pain may be achieved by sitting up or leaning forward. In addition, there may be a history of prodromal symptoms which can include fever, malaise and myalgia. In mild cases, signs may be absent; however, there may be signs of dyspnoea, raised JVP, Kussmaul's sign, pulsus paradoxus, systemic hypotension and diminished heart sounds.

Investigations

Haematological indices may show a raised WBC and ESR, but these are non-specific. Cardiac enzymes may be elevated if the inflammation extends to the surface myocardium. Other specific haematological/serological investigations may be necessary to confirm a suspected aetiology (see Table 22.1).

An ECG must be performed to exclude an acute MI. In acute

Table 22.1 Causes of pericarditis.

Infections:	Viral, e.g. Coxsackie B, echovirus, HIV
	Bacterial, e.g. staphylococci, streptococci,
	  Haemophilus influenzae, meningococcus,
	  salmonella, psittacosis,
	  tuberculosis, syphilis
	  Mycoplasma pneumoniae
	Fungal, e.g. histoplasmosis, aspergillosis
	Others, e.g. rickettsiae, amoebiasis, echinococcus

Neoplasms:	Primary, e.g. mesothelioma, angiosarcoma,
	  teratoma, fibroma
	Secondary, e.g. lung, breast, leukaemia,
	  lymphoma, melanoma, Kaposi's sarcoma, colon

Connective tissue disease:	e.g. SLE, rheumatic fever, rheumatoid arthritis, polyarteritis nodosa
Drug induced:	e.g. hydralizine, procainamide, dantrolene, daunorubicin
Post-myocardial injury:	e.g. post-MI, Dressler's syndrome, trauma, post- surgical, radiation
Other:	e.g. uraemia, myxoedema, sarcoidosis

pericarditis, it typically shows widespread ST segment elevation (concave upwards). After several days, widespread T-wave inversion may occur.

In most cases a CXR will be normal, but cardiac enlargement suggests possible pericardial effusion. If this is suspected, echocardiography will be necessary to confirm the presence of an effusion and monitor its progress.

Management

Initially supportive care, whilst other more life-threatening conditions are excluded. Specific therapy consists of non-steroidal anti-inflammatory agents (e.g. ibuprofen, aspirin). If these fail, a short course of steroids may be of benefit.

Patients with uraemic pericarditis need to be considered for intensive dialysis therapy. Other aetiologies of pericarditis will require specific therapy for the underlying disorder. Patients with symptomatic effusions or tamponade will require pericardial aspiration (See Chapter 23).

Cardiac tamponade

Background

Cardiac tamponade occurs when blood or other fluid fills the pericardial space, raising intrapericardial pressure, compressing the heart and preventing it from filling. As the heart is unable to fill adequately, stroke volume, blood pressure and cardiac output decrease, and signs of shock with a raised venous pressure develop. Tamponade and death can occur with only a few hundred millilitres of effusion, if it develops rapidly; conversely, it may take in excess of a litre of effusion to produce tamponade if it accumulates over a long period of time.

There are many possible causes of cardiac tamponade. The commonest seen in CCU is rupture of the free wall of the ventricle following acute infarction, which is usually rapidly fatal. Occasionally, a patient will be seen who develops tamponade following cardiac catheterization or temporary pacing. Malignant pericardial effusions causing tamponade are not unusual, but tend to have a less acute presentation. There should be a high index of suspicion that tamponade is present in a haemodynamically collapsed patient with renal failure, post-cardiac surgery, and following chest injuries (particularly in patients treated with anticoagulants).

Clinical presentation

The major clinical signs of tamponade are:
1. Hypotension with pulsus paradoxus
2. Raised venous pressure with positive Kussmaul's sign
3. Soft heart sounds. There may be a pericardial rub.

The ECG may show electrical alternans and low voltage QRS complexes, whilst a globular heart may be seen on the CXR. The best way to make a definitive diagnosis is by echocardiography. Treatment of a large effusion causing tamponade is by pericardiocentesis, described in Chapter 23. If you suspect tamponade, contact a senior colleague for advice on pericardiocentesis.

Myocardial contusion

The incidence of this condition appears to depend on how eagerly it is sought. It occurs as a result of blunt trauma, commonly from steering wheel injury. Sub-epicardial bruising is the usual pathological finding, although in more severe injury there is bruising into the myocardium. The key symptom is chest pain, typically unrelieved by nitrates. There may also be inappropriate tachycardia, gallop rhythm and pericardial rub. The clinical findings are generally overshadowed by other injuries. The ECG may show non-specific ST segment and T-wave changes compatible with acute pericarditis, and rhythm changes are common. Pathological Q-waves may develop after severe injury. Cardiac enzymes are often elevated, and echocardiography may show regional wall motion abnormalities. Treatment is initially with analgesia and bed rest, although any of the complications of myocardial infarction may develop. Complete recovery is the rule, as patients are often young with an otherwise healthy heart.

Infective endocarditis

Background

Overall there are approximately 1500 cases of endocarditis in the UK per year, with approximately 15 per cent mortality. It is now well accepted that infective endocarditis can occur on a previously healthy valve, although any congenital or acquired structural cardiac abnormality will increase an individual's risk. Generally, turbulent blood flow from a high to low pressure zone will damage the endocardium, resulting in a sterile platelet–fibrin thrombus. An episode of bacteraemia may then seed this thrombus, proliferating and resulting in infective endocarditis. Typical portals of entry for the bacteraemia include:

1. Dental work
2. Genitourinary infection/instrumentation
3. IV drug abuse
4. Surgery
5. IV cannulation
6. Endoscopy procedures.

Individuals at particularly high risk include those who are immunocompromised, and those who have prosthetic heart valves or chronic medical conditions such as diabetes, renal failure and alcoholism. As with all medical conditions, prevention is better than cure, so any patient with structural heart disease undergoing an 'at risk' medical/dental procedure should have antibiotic prophylaxis.

Organisms commonly responsible for infective endocarditis include:

1. *Streptococcus viridans* group (e.g. *S. milleri, S. mutans, S. mitis, S. mitior, S. bovis*)
2. Staphylococci (e.g. *S. aureus, S. epidermidis*)
3. Enterococci group (e.g. *S. faecalis*).

Other rarer bacterial infections can also be responsible, such as gram-negative bacilli, diphtheroids and acid-fast bacilli. Non-bacterial infections include fungi, rickettsiae, *Coxiella burnetii* and chlamydiae.

Diagnosis

In a susceptible individual, consideration of the diagnosis is vital as the physical signs may mimic many other medical conditions. In particular there may be evidence of a generalized infection, the signs of which include fever, pallor, rigors, night sweats, malaise, weight loss, splenomegaly and clubbing. There may also be signs of embolic or immunologic phenomena, which include splinter haemorrhages, Janeway lesions, Osler's nodes, conjunctival petechiae and Roth spots. Classically there is a new or changing cardiac murmur, and in severe cases (when complications develop) there may be arrhythmias, heart block (suggestive of abscess formation), increasing valvular regurgitation and cardiac failure.

Investigations

1. Blood cultures are paramount for diagnosis and monitoring treatment. Three sets of cultures (aerobic and anaerobic) containing at least 10 ml of blood should be taken from different sites, at different times, and before the commencement of antibiotics.
2. FBC, ESR. These may show anaemia, raised white cell count and high ESR. CRP is useful for monitoring therapy.
3. Microscopy/MSU may show haematuria.
4. ECG – no specific changes, but this may reveal the development of complications (e.g. lengthening PR interval).
5. CXR. This may show signs of heart failure or pulmonary infiltrates from septic emboli.
6. Swabs, taken from skin lesions, cannulation sites, nasal cavity.
7. Echocardiography. A transthoracic scan may identify vegetations and valvular dysfunction. A transoesophageal scan has greater diagnostic yield and is better for detecting complications such as an aortic root abscess.
8. Antibody titres for unusual organisms, if bacterial cultures are negative.

Treatment

If the diagnosis is suspected and cultures have been taken, then intravenous antibiotics should be commenced. Intravenous lines should be re-sited regularly, to reduce further risk of infection. There are no hard and fast rules for the duration of therapy; this will depend on the sensitivity of the organisms and the patient's response to and tolerance of treatment. Close liaison with the microbiologist is essential to guide antibiotic therapy and monitor peak/trough antibiotic levels. A bactericidal antibiotic is essential. The following suggestions are for guidance for initial therapy only, as local practices will vary.

Strep. viridans	IV benzyl penicillin and/or gentamicin
Staph. aureus	IV flucloxacillin, fucidic acid and gentamicin
Gram negatives	IV ampicillin, gentamicin and/or metronidazole (for anaerobic infection)
Enterococci	IV benzyl penicillin and gentamicin
Fungi	IV amphotericin B
Coxiella burnetii	doxycycline, rifampicin

Anticoagulation is no longer used routinely, due to the risk of haemorrhage at a potential site of embolus impaction, unless there is another medical indication (e.g. prosthetic valve, DVT, pulmonary embolus, atrial fibrillation).

Surgical intervention

This is generally indicated after failed medical therapy (e.g. relapse after treatment or fungal infection), or when complications develop. Progressive valvular regurgitation, refractory heart failure, intracardiac abscess formation, major systemic emboli and large mobile vegetations are all indications for surgical intervention.

Digoxin toxicity

Digoxin is commonly used to control chronic atrial fibrillation and heart failure. However, high plasma levels can lead to symptoms of toxicity and cardiac arrhythmias. Typical symptoms of toxicity include:

1. Anorexia, nausea, vomiting

2. Confusion, fits, paraesthesiae
3. Visual disturbance (e.g. blurring, xanthopsia).

High plasma levels of digoxin are most likely to occur in the setting of hypokalaemia, hypercalcaemia and hypomagnesaemia. In addition, toxicity is more likely to occur in patients who are elderly, have impaired renal function, or are taking medication known to increase plasma digoxin levels. Drugs known to increase plasma digoxin include quinidine, captopril, amiodarone, propafenone, verapamil, nifedipine, erythromycin and tetracycline.

The dose of digoxin should be reduced in patients who are susceptible to toxicity. The commonest ECG change seen in digoxin toxicity is atrial tachycardia with AV block. Other abnormalities include junctional bradycardia, ventricular bigeminy, ventricular ectopics/salvos, paroxysmal VT and second or third degree AV block.

If you suspect digoxin toxicity:

1. Stop digoxin
2. Correct hypokalaemia if present
3. Monitor cardiac rhythm and correct any sustained haemodynamically significant arrhythmia that occurs
4. Check digoxin levels. A serum digoxin level of greater than 3.5 mmol/l supports the clinical diagnosis.

Treatment is with beta-blockers if the ventricular rate is fast (as detailed in Chapter 8). Phenytoin by slow IV injection was formerly used to control ventricular arrhythmias caused by cardiac glycosides, but this is now obsolete.

Remember to avoid DC cardioversion for the treatment of tachyarrhythmias in a patient with digoxin toxicity, as it may induce intractable arrhythmias. If you have to give a DC shock as a last resort, start at a low energy level (i.e. 10 joules). In the treatment of digoxin overdose, treatment with digoxin antibody fragments (digibind) in addition to the above measures may be life saving.

Tricyclic antidepressant overdose

Tricyclic antidepressants result in a significant mortality when taken in overdose due to the cardiac effects of hypotension and arrhythmia. Most life-threatening events occur within six hours of ingestion. Initially, anticholinergic signs predominate (dilated pupils, warm dry skin, dry mouth, decreased bowel sounds, sedation and tachycardia), which may then rapidly progress to bradycardia, heart block and asystole in cases of serious overdose. Hypotension accompanies the decreased cardiac output, and there may be a decrease in mental status, respiratory depression and seizures. As tricyclics interfere with the movement of sodium ions, all intervals on the ECG are prolonged. Classically the effect is on the QRS complex, and if its duration is greater than 120 ms this is a good predictor of cardiac and neurological toxicity. A QRS complex duration of greater than 160 ms is predictive of dysrhythmias.

Management is generally supportive, with monitoring of respiration and cardiac rhythm. Owing to the possibility of rapid deterioration, gastric lavage and instillation of activated charcoal are recommended. Noradrenaline is the vasopressor of choice, although dobutamine may be effective in the presence of a low cardiac output but adequate filling pressures. Acidosis can aggravate the cardiotoxicity of tricyclics; correcting this with sodium bicarbonate can reduce the prolongation of the ECG and help correct hypotension and arrhythmias. For seizures, benzodiazepines are the drug of choice (phenytoin may aggravate cardiac arrhythmias). If seizures cannot be adequately controlled, paralysis and ventilation are indicated to prevent further acidosis.

Key points

- Consider pericardial tamponade in a haemodynamically collapsed patient who has risk factors.

- In cases of infective endocarditis, three blood cultures should be taken before IV antibiotics are commenced.

- Consider digoxin toxicity in any patients on digoxin therapy, particularly if they are dehydrated, hypokalaemic or have unusual arrhythmias.

- Tricyclic overdose is common and potentially fatal, usually within the first six hours of ingestion. The ECG is the best guide to cardiotoxicity.

References

Aldridge, J. and Wilson, R. (1998). Dental health and the cardiovascular patient. *Br. J. Cardiol.*, **5**, 28–34.

Anderson, D. R. (1993). The diagnosis and management of non-penetrating cardiothoracic trauma. *Br. J. Clin. Pract.*, **47**, 97–103.

British Society for Antimicrobial Chemotherapy. (1990). Antibiotic prophylaxis of infective endocarditis: recommendations from the Endocarditis Working Party. *Lancet*, **335**, 88–89.

Leader. (1976). Sodium bicarbonate and tricyclic antidepressant poisoning. *Lancet*, **ii**, 838.

Spodick, D. H. (1983). The normal and diseased pericardium: current concepts of pericardial physiology, diagnosis and treatment. *J. Am. Coll. Cardiol.*, **1**, 240–251.

Verhaul, H. A., Van den Brink, R. B., Van Vreeland, T., *et al.* (1993). Effects of changes in management of active infective endocarditis on outcome in a 25 year period. *Am. J. Cardiol.*, **72**, 682–687.

23

Practical procedures

No written guidelines can replace instruction by an experienced colleague. These short notes are meant to be used as an adjunct to this, and not as a replacement for it.

Central venous cannulation

Cannulation of a central vein is used on CCU in order to:

1. Monitor central cardiac pressures and cardiac output to guide therapy
2. Insert temporary pacing wires
3. Provide a route for administration of drugs, such as dopamine, that should not be given via a peripheral line
4. Provide IV access in a patient with no suitable peripheral veins.

A number of sites can be used to provide central venous access. In general, the right subclavian vein is recommended unless the patient has a bleeding tendency (e.g. liver disease, warfarin or recent thrombolytic therapy), in which case the internal jugular vein, antecubital fossa veins or the femoral venous route are preferred, since these allow easier haemostasis to be achieved.

Subclavian cannulation using a Seldinger (needle and guidewire) technique

1. Explain the procedure to the patient.
2. Lie the patient flat, with a head down tilt if possible (this facilitates venous filling and reduces the risk of air embolism). Slightly rotate the patient's head to the opposite side.
3. Operator scrubs, and sterile gloves and gown are worn.
4. Clean and drape the skin.
5. Infiltrate local anaesthetic below the junction of the medial one-third

and lateral two-thirds of the clavicle, and nick the skin at this point with a scalpel blade.

6. Straighten the clavicle by having an assistant apply gentle traction to the patient's right arm.

7. Place your left index finger in the suprasternal notch, and advance the introducer needle from the skin nick towards your finger until you come into contact with the clavicle. Move the tip of the needle down until it lies just below the clavicle, then slowly advance the needle towards your finger in the suprasternal notch whilst continuously aspirating for blood. Avoid pointing the tip of the needle downwards to minimize the risk of an iatrogenic pneumothorax.

8. When the vein is punctured, remove the syringe, cover the needle with your thumb to prevent the entry of air and insert the guide wire flexible end first. The wire should enter freely with no resistance. If you encounter resistance, remove the wire and check that the tip of the needle is still in the vein by aspirating more blood, then try again. Never force the wire against resistance.

9. When the guide wire is in place, remove the needle. Depending on equipment, either make a tract with the dilator first and then insert the cannula over the wire or insert the dilator and cannula as a single unit, using a rotating motion. Always make sure the tip of the guide wire is visible at all times. Finally, remove the wire, leaving the cannula in place.

10. Secure the cannula with a suture, and cover with a sterile porous dressing.

11. Check a post-procedure CXR to exclude pneumothorax and confirm line position.

Internal jugular cannulation

This has gained in popularity, as there is less risk of iatrogenic pneumothorax or arterial puncture. The right side is easier to cannulate than the left, and the area of the thoracic duct is avoided. However, this may not be the ideal site for elective cannulation if access is required for several days (e.g. temporary pacing wires), due to difficulties in securing the catheter.

Anatomy

The internal jugular vein emerges from the base of the skull between the mastoid process and the angle of the jaw. It passes deep to the sternomastoid and omohyoid muscles, and runs in the carotid sheath lateral to the internal and common carotid arteries. It joins the subclavian vein behind the sternal end of the clavicle to form the brachio-cephalic vein.

Insertion

1. Explain the procedure to the patient.

2. Lie the patient flat, with a head down tilt if possible (this facilitates venous filling and reduces the risk of air embolism). Slightly rotate the patient's head to the opposite side.

3. Operator scrubs, and sterile gloves and gown are worn.

4. Clean and drape the skin.

5. Infiltrate local anaesthetic into the skin over the sternomastoid muscle, just medial to the line of the vein in the middle of its course. Infiltrate the deeper structures in the direction of the vein.

6. Using a syringe and fine needle, locate the vein by continuous aspiration. This can be left in position as a guide.

7. The Seldinger needle is inserted into the internal jugular vein at an angle of 30° to the skin, with the tip of the needle directed towards the ipsilateral nipple. With continuous aspiration, blood will enter the syringe when the vein is punctured.

8. When the vein is punctured, remove the syringe, cover the needle with your thumb to prevent the entry of air and insert the guide wire flexible end first. The wire should enter freely with no resistance. If you encounter resistance, remove the wire and check that the tip of the needle is still in the vein by aspirating more blood, then try again. Never force the wire against resistance.

9. When the guide wire is in place, remove the needle. Depending on equipment, either make a tract with the dilator first and then insert the cannula over the wire or insert the dilator and cannula as a single unit, using a rotating motion. Always make sure the tip of the guide wire is visible at all times. Finally, remove the wire, leaving the cannula in place.

10. Secure the cannula with a suture, and cover with a sterile porous dressing.

11. Check a post-procedure CXR to exclude pneumothorax and confirm line position.

Key points

- Choose the correct puncture site.
- Do not hesitate to seek assistance from a senior colleague.
- After failed subclavian puncture, obtain a CXR *before* attempting contralateral catheterization.

Temporary pacing

Temporary pacing is a necessary skill for all junior doctors managing acute medical patients. The general indications for temporary pacing are actual or threatened bradycardia due to conduction tissue disease, procedures associated with important bradycardia, or overdrive suppression of malignant ventricular arrhythmias. However, there are no categorical rules about the need for temporary pacing and the decision should be made by an experienced doctor. In particular, the potential complications of the procedure may outweigh the benefits when considering prophylactic temporary pacing.

Procedure

1. Before starting, ensure that the resuscitation trolley is easily accessible and that you have venous access to give drugs if necessary. Brady- or tachyarrhythmias are often induced during the procedure, so ensure that atropine, isoprenaline and lignocaine are readily at hand should they be needed. In an emergency, external transthoracic pacing (if available) can provide short-term support until a temporary wire can be inserted.

2. The best route for placing a temporary wire is usually via the right subclavian vein (the left side is then available for a permanent implant if required). If subclavian puncture is contraindicated (e.g. thrombolysis), use the femoral or internal jugular; these have the advantage that haemostasis can easily be secured by pressure if bleeding occurs.

3. A sheath with a non-return valve should be placed in the vein using a Seldinger technique, to allow easy manipulation of the wire (see central venous cannulation). Strict surgical asepsis should be followed at all times.

4. A size 5F or 6F bipolar pacing wire is appropriate in most cases. Ensure that a working pacing box (pulse generator) is ready before inserting the wire.

5. With a 20–30° curve at the wire tip, advance the wire into the right atrium under fluoroscopic control and rotate until it points downwards and to the patient's left. Advancing across the tricuspid valve will often induce arrhythmias, which usually settle rapidly and require no treatment. If difficulty is encountered in crossing the tricuspid valve, changing the curve at the wire tip usually helps. If this fails, try fashioning the electrode into a loop in the right atrium and manoeuvring it across the valve by twisting it one way or the other.

6. The best position for the pacing wire is usually with the tip in the right ventricular apex, to the left of the midline and with the tip of the wire pointing inferiorly on screening (if the wire is directed to the left and upwards, it may be in the coronary sinus and often will not capture at an acceptable threshold).

7. To test the threshold, set the pacing rate at 5–10 bpm faster than the patient's rate, and turn the amplitude of the voltage down until capture is lost. Acceptable stimulation thresholds are below one volt, although higher levels may be acceptable if the patient is elderly, has had an inferior infarct, or if several sites have been tried all with relatively high thresholds.

8. To check the stability of the pacing wire, pace at an output twice the threshold during deep breathing. If capture is lost during this manoeuvre, then try to find a more stable position.

9. Remember to suture the wire firmly with a loop formed on the chest wall to minimize the chance of inadvertent displacement.

10. The pacing threshold should be checked twice daily, and a sudden increase in the threshold usually indicates the need for repositioning. Pacing thresholds are checked by increasing the pacing rate to obtain continuous pacing, then progressively decreasing the output voltage until capture is lost. The minimum output voltage which provides consistent capture is the pacing threshold voltage. Once the threshold has been ascertained, the output voltage should be set at three times the threshold to ensure a margin of safety.

Pulmonary artery catheterization

Pulmonary artery balloon flotation catheters enable central cardiac pressures and cardiac output to be monitored. This information can be very useful in diagnosis and treatment, but placement of these lines is not without risk of complications, either related to insertion (e.g. pneumothorax, arrhythmia, pulmonary artery rupture) or to maintenance of an indwelling foreign body (e.g. infection, thrombosis). The procedure should, therefore, only be carried out if the information provided will be of definite benefit to the patient.

Indications for use

1. Low output states post-MI. These may be due to cardiogenic shock, hypovolaemia, right ventricular infarction or ruptured ventricular septum. Measurement of cardiac haemodynamics will enable differentiation of these conditions, and therefore appropriate treatment.

2. Differential diagnosis of pulmonary oedema. In cardiogenic pulmonary oedema there will be a raised pulmonary artery wedge pressure, whereas with other causes of diffuse alveolar shadowing (e.g. adult respiratory distress syndrome) the wedge pressure is low or normal.

Placement of the catheter

1. Calibrate the catheter by positioning the pressure transducer at mid-axillary level with the patient supine, and pressing the zero button on the pressure monitor.

2. Insert a suitable central venous sheath.

3. Check balloon by inflating with saline before insertion.

4. Flush the catheter with saline, connect to the monitoring system, and check that pressure is being recorded by moving the tip of the catheter rapidly up and down and observing the simultaneous deflections of the pressure trace.

5. Insert the catheter 10 cm (circumferential lines on the catheter are 10 cm apart) and inflate the balloon. Advance the catheter (using x-ray guidance) to the pulmonary artery (it should float easily into position when the balloon is inflated). If x-ray guidance is not available, observation of the pressure trace can be used to guide catheter placement (Figure 23.1). However, do not attempt to place a catheter without x-ray guidance unless you have done so before, under supervision.

6. Ventricular arrhythmias (usually runs of ectopics) are common as the catheter crosses the tricuspid valve.

7. When a wedge trace is acquired, deflate the balloon. A phasic pulmonary artery trace should reappear; if it does not, the catheter should be withdrawn slightly and the balloon reinflated and deflated until it is possible to obtain both a wedge and phasic pulmonary artery trace with the balloon fully inflated and then deflated. The catheter is now in an optimal position.

8. The catheter should not be left wedged after measurements have been made, as this may lead to pulmonary infarction.

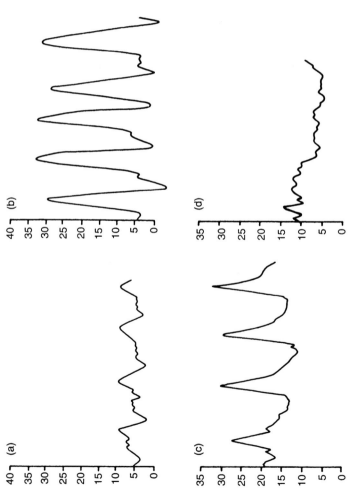

Figure 23.1 Normal intracardiac pressure tracings obtained as a pulmonary artery catheter passes through the right heart. (a) = right atrium; (b) = right ventricle; (c) = pulmonary artery; and (d) = mean wedge pressure.

Additional information

1. In addition to the pressure measurements that can be made as the catheter is advanced through the right heart, it is also possible to take intracardiac blood samples. After discarding the first 2 ml of blood from the catheter, samples can be collected in heparinized syringes for assessment of oxygen saturation. If an oxygen step up is found between the SVC and PA, then further samples can be taken to localize the shunt more precisely. A large step up in saturation from one chamber to the next implies the presence of a large defect, and substantial left to right shunt.

2. For thermodilution studies, the thermistors are attached to the cardiac output computer. A closed system is used, which allows the injection of iced saline through the proximal port of the catheter. After each injection, the computer estimates the cardiac output. Three or more reproducible estimates should be averaged to obtain the working figures.

Potential problems

1. Pressure trace damped. This is due to kinking of the catheter, air bubbles in the pressure monitor, thrombus occluding the catheter tip or the catheter being sited too far into the pulmonary artery, and can usually be solved by checking the pressure monitoring system for bubbles or kinks, flushing the catheter, or withdrawing the catheter a few centimetres.

2. Failure to wedge. This is due to the catheter being placed too proximally, or to balloon rupture. If the balloon ruptures, blood will collect in the inflation syringe and the catheter should be replaced if continued monitoring of the wedge pressure is necessary. Advancing the catheter a few centimetres will enable a wedge trace to be obtained visually if the catheter is sited too proximally.

3. Whenever possible do not leave a catheter *in situ* for more than 48 hours, to minimize the risk of infection. If infection occurs, remove the catheter, take blood cultures, and treat initially with broad spectrum IV antibiotics.

Normal range of intracardiac pressure (measured from mid-chest).

Site	Pressure (mmHg)
RA	0–7
RV	15–25/0–8
PA	15–25/8–15
PAWP	6–12

NB: Wedge pressure is normally measured at end expiration. In a patient with COPD, pressures may be falsely elevated. In a patient without COPD, pulmonary artery diastolic pressure is normally equivalent to the wedge pressure.

Pericardial aspiration

Pericardial effusion causing tamponade is a life-threatening condition. Typical signs may include tachycardia, hypotension, raised JVP, tachypnoea, quiet heart sounds, pericardial rub and/or fever. The CXR classically shows a large globular heart in the absence of pulmonary congestion. The ECG may show small complexes, electrical alternans or concave ST elevation. Pericardial aspiration is indicated in patients with haemodynamic compromise, in which case it may be life saving. It is also performed occasionally for diagnostic purposes. It should be remembered that pericardial aspiration is a potentially dangerous procedure; only attempt it if a senior colleague is available to supervise. Guidelines for pericardial aspiration are set out below:

1. Pericardial aspiration should ideally be performed with full x-ray screening, rhythm monitoring and resuscitation facilities readily available. If available, echocardiography can be used to guide pericardial aspiration, since it allows you to visualize the fluid filled space, the myocardium and the aspiration needle. It can therefore give an indication of the best line of approach.

2. Place the patient at 30–45° (to pool the pericardial fluid inferiorly). Connect the patient to an ECG monitor.

3. Connect the V1 lead from the ECG machine via a clip to the aspiration needle. If you touch the myocardium with the needle, ST elevation will immediately show on the monitor, giving you warning to stop advancing the needle.

4. Clean the skin and maintain an aseptic technique. Infiltrate lignocaine

below and to the left of the xiphoid process. The subxiphoid approach is usually preferable, as it is extrapleural and avoids the internal mammary arteries.

5. Advance the needle towards the left shoulder, aspirating as you do so. Stop if ST elevation develops on the monitor, or as soon as you aspirate pericardial fluid or when the needle is seen to enter the pericardial space on the echocardiogram.

6. Insert a guide wire under radiological or ultrasound control, predilate and insert a pigtail drainage catheter over the wire. Remove the wire and leave the catheter *in situ*, connected to a collection bag if there is any possibility of the fluid reaccumulating.

7. The pericardial fluid should be sent to microbiology (microscopy, culture and sensitivity), biochemistry (protein, glucose) and cytology.

8. The catheter is generally removed after 24–48 hours, to reduce the chance of infection. Recurrent effusions may require the formation of a pericardial window, a balloon pericardiotomy or the installation of chemotherapeutic agents.

DC cardioversion

DC cardioversion can be performed as an elective procedure, for chronic arrhythmias which have failed to revert with drug therapy, or when drugs have not been tolerated or are contraindicated. Urgent DC cardioversion is indicated for arrhythmias which are causing acute hypotension, heart failure or ischaemia.

In elective cases, the patient's status should be optimized prior to the procedure. Full oral anticoagulation with warfarin is necessary for at least one month before the procedure, unless the arrhythmia is of very recent onset (< 24 hours) or transoesophageal echocardiography (TOE) has been used to exclude thrombi or spontaneous echo contrast in the atria. In addition, metabolic abnormalities or hypoxia should be corrected and medication reviewed (digoxin need not be withheld provided toxicity is excluded). At present it is recommended that all patients receive warfarin for at least four weeks following DC cardioversion, although this strategy is currently under investigation.

DC cardioversion should be avoided if digoxin toxicity is present, as it may induce refractory ventricular arrhythmias or asystole. Lignocaine, phenytoin, beta-blockers and overdrive pacing can all be used to treat digoxin-induced arrhythmias.

The following procedure should generally be followed:

1. The patient should be fasted, have consented, and have IV access *in situ.*
2. Electrolytes and anticoagulation should have been checked.
3. A general anaesthetic is preferable in elective cases; however, for urgent cardioversion (if consciousness is not lost as a result of the arrhythmia) the patient should be sedated with 5–10 mg of intravenous diazepam.
4. Conductive gel or pads should be used in conjunction with firm pressure on the chest wall, so as to reduce transthoracic impedance.
5. A synchronized shock should be used in all arrhythmias except VF.
6. In general, the lowest possible initial energy should be utilized in order to minimize the risk of cardiac damage. Low energies may suffice in supraventricular arrhythmias (particularly atrial flutter), and 25 joules may be successful. For atrial fibrillation or ventricular tachycardia, the suggested initial energy level is 100 J.
7. If initial attempts at cardioversion fail, try moving the paddles to the apex–posterior position (so that one paddle is over the apex and the other is below the right scapula to the right of the spine).

Key points

- Obtain instruction and supervision from an experienced colleague in all practical procedures.
- If placement of a central venous line proves difficult, do not persist in your attempts – ask a senior colleague for help.
- Pulmonary artery catheters are most useful in hypotensive patients. However, their use is not without complications, and a definite indication for use should be present. The majority of patients with post-MI heart failure will not benefit from insertion of a pulmonary artery catheter.
- All patients requiring elective DC cardioversion should be anti-coagulated for one month prior to and following the procedure.

References

Chin, D. T. and Robinson, N. M. (1995). How to catheterize the right heart. *Brit. J. Cardiol.*, **2(9)**, 255–259.

Connors, A., Speroff, T., Dawson, N., *et al.* (1996). The effectiveness of right heart catheterization in the initial care of critically ill patients. *JAMA*, **276**, 889–897.

Ewy, G. A. (1994). The optimal technique for electrical cardioversion of atrial fibrillation. *Clin. Cardiol.*, **17**, 79–84.

Hehir, D. J., Stansby, G., Stuart, R. C., *et al.* (1992). Catheterization of the subclavian vein. *Hospital Update*, 295–299.

Krikorian, J. G. and Hancock, E. W. (1978). Pericardiocentesis. *Am. J. Med.*, **65**, 808–814.

Manning, W. J., Silverman, D. I., Gordon, S. P. F., *et al.* (1993). Cardioversion from atrial fibrillation without prolonged anticoagulation with use of transesophogeal echocardiography to exclude the presence of atrial thrombi. *N. Engl. J. Med.*, **328**, 750–755.

Rothman, M. T. (1981). Temporary cardiac pacing. *Hosp. Update*, **7**, 645–652.

24

Intravenous cardiac drugs

This chapter provides brief information on commonly used intravenous cardiac drugs, in particular those agents used in resuscitation or those requiring continuous infusion. It is not meant to be a comprehensive list, but rather a rapid source of information. It must be stressed that indications, contraindications and administration may change over the course of time; if in doubt, always check with an up-to-date edition of the *British National Formulary* (BNF).

Adenosine

Indication: First line therapy for AVNRT.

A rapid IV bolus into large peripheral vein, flushed through with 10 ml saline. Initial dose 3 mg, followed by incremental doses of 6 mg and 12 mg at one to two minute intervals.

NB: Dipyridamole potentiates the effect of adenosine.

Adrenaline

Indication: For cardiac arrest.

10 ml of a 1:10 000 mini-jet (1 mg) IV, repeated as per resuscitation guidelines.

Indication: For inotropic support.

5 ml of a 1:1000 injection in 50 ml 5% dextrose or normal saline (100 mg/ml). Infuse at 0.5 to 15 ml/hr, depending on response (0.01 to 0.5 mcg/kg/min).

Indication: For anaphylaxis.

0.5 to 1.0 ml of a 1:1000 mini-jet IM. If there is doubt as to the adequacy of the circulation, give adrenaline by slow intravenous injection – 5 ml of a 1:10 000 injection IV at a rate of 100 micrograms (1 ml) per minute, stopping when a response has been obtained.

Alteplase (Actilyse, rt-PA)

Indication: Accelerated regime for acute MI.

15 mg IV bolus, followed by 0.75 mg/kg (to a maximum of 50 mg) over 30 minutes, then 0.5 mg/kg (to a maximum of 35 mg) over 60 minutes. Give 5000 U of heparin IV as a bolus before starting rt-PA administration, then after completion of the rt-PA infusion give 1,00 U/hr (adjusted according to APTT after six hours).

Indication: Pulmonary embolism.

10 mg by IV injection over one to two minutes, followed by 90 mg as an infusion over two hours. Heparin should be given as a 5000 U bolus at the start of the rt-PA infusion, followed by an infusion commenced at the end of the rt-PA infusion (adjusted to maintain the APTT 2–3 times the control value).

Amiodarone

Indication: For treatment of ventricular or supraventricular arrhythmias.

5 mg/kg in 100 ml 5% dextrose (do *not* use normal saline) over 20 minutes, followed by an infusion of 900 mg in 500 ml 5% dextrose over 24 hours, repeated as clinically indicated. Maximum recommended dose is 1.2 g amiodarone in 24 hours. Administration via a central line is preferable to avoid thrombophlebitis if a prolonged infusion is required. A peripheral line (large arm vein) is acceptable for 24 hours in a post-infarction patient. Oral dose is usually 200 mg tds for one week, 200 mg bd for one week, reducing to maintenance dose of 50–200 mg daily.

NB: Amiodarone potentiates digoxin and warfarin. It is pro-arrhythmic, particularly at the start of therapy. Monitor liver and thyroid function in patients on long-term therapy.

Atropine

Indication: For use in sinus bradycardia.

0.3 to 1.0 mg IV repeated every three to five minutes to a total of

0.04 mg/kg body weight. Side-effects include tachycardia, dry mouth, difficult visual accommodation, hesitant micturition and constipation.

Indication: For resuscitation.

3 mg bolus (mini-jet) as per resuscitation guidelines.

Bretylium tosylate

Indication: For short-term control of ventricular arrhythmias resistant to standard treatment during resuscitation.

A delay of half an hour or more can occur before the onset of antiarrhythmic activity. It may cause severe hypotension, which should be corrected using a plasma volume expander. Give 5 to 10 mg/kg body weight by slow intravenous injection (dilute to 10 mg/ml using 5% dextrose or normal saline before administration). Nausea and vomiting may occur, and this can be avoided by giving the injection over not less than eight minutes, although 15 to 30 minutes is preferred. The IV injection can be repeated in one to two hours if the arrhythmia persists. An IV infusion in 5% dextrose at 1–2 mg/minute can be used as an alternative to bolus dosing.

Calcium chloride/gluconate

Indications: For EMD arrest, hyperkalaemia, hypocalcaemia and calcium antagonist toxicity.

10 ml 10% solution slowly IV. *Do not* use the same line as for sodium bicarbonate infusion.

Digibind

Indication: For the treatment of life-threatening manifestations of intoxication by digoxin or digitoxin.

Reserve for use in patients where digoxin withdrawal and correction of electrolyte abnormalities are felt to be insufficient (see Chapter 22). Contact unit pharmacist or on-call pharmacist immediately to order digibind into the hospital. For dosage instructions refer to company data sheet.

Digoxin

Indications: For management of AF, and for inotropic support in heart failure.

A loading dose is not required for use in mild heart failure. In the management of AF, patients should be orally loaded as follows:

1. 250–500 mcg eight hourly for 24 hours
2. 125–250 mcg daily thereafter.

Lower loading and maintenance doses may be sufficient in older patients, or those with renal impairment. It is important to ensure that serum potassium is above 4.0 mmol/l when administering digoxin, as hypokalaemia will potentiate toxic side-effects. The maintenance dose is governed by ventricular response, which should normally be maintained above 60 bpm. Loading dose should be given IV only if the patient is nil by mouth or vomiting – there is no advantage to this route. Give in 100 ml 5% dextrose or normal saline over two to four hours (too rapid an administration is associated with nausea and risk of arrhythmias). If a rapid effect is desired, other agents or DC cardioversion may be more appropriate. For plasma concentration monitoring, blood should ideally be taken at least six hours after a dose.

Dobutamine

Indications: Inotropic support in infarction, cardiac surgery, septic and cardiogenic shock.

250 mg in 50 ml 5% dextrose or normal saline gives a drug concentration of 5000 mcg/ml. This can be given via a peripheral line. Infuse at 2.5 mcg/kg/min initially, increasing to a maximum of 20 mcg/kg/min. The following table gives infusion rates in millilitres per hour for a solution of 5000 mcg/ml according to dose required and body weight.

		Body weight (kg)				
		50	60	70	80	90
Dobutamine	2.5	1.5	1.8	2.1	2.4	2.7
infusion rate	5.0	3.0	3.6	4.2	4.8	5.4
(mcg/kg/min)	10	6.0	7.2	8.4	9.6	10.8
	15	9.0	10.8	12.6	15.4	16.2
	20	12.0	14.4	16.8	19.2	21.6

Dopamine

At low (2.5 mcg/kg/min) infusion rates, dopamine acts selectively on renal dopamine receptors to cause vasodilatation and increased renal blood flow, and it is therefore useful in oliguric patients with low cardiac output. At higher doses (above 5 mcg/kg/min), dopamine acts on alpha receptors to produce vasoconstriction and may therefore be useful in a patient with persistent hypotension. It should only be given via a central line, since extravasation from a peripheral line may cause severe ischaemic injury due to vasoconstriction.

Add 400 mg (in 10 ml) to 40 ml 5% dextrose to give a total volume of 50 ml, and a drug concentration of 8000 mcg/ml. Infuse at 2.5–5.0 mcg/kg/min to produce optimal renal vasodilatation. Infuse at 5–20 mcg/kg/min to support a low blood pressure by producing systemic vasoconstriction. The following table gives infusion rates in ml/hr for an 8000 mcg/ml solution according to dose required and body weight.

		Body weight (kg)				
		50	60	70	80	90
Dopamine	2.5	0.9	1.1	1.3	1.5	1.7
infusion rate	5.0	1.9	2.3	2.6	3.0	3.4
(mcg/kg/min)	10	3.8	4.5	5.2	6.0	6.8
	15	5.7	6.8	7.8	9.0	10.2
	20	7.6	9.0	10.4	12.0	13.6

Esmolol

Indication: For acute management of SVT (including AF and atrial flutter).

This is a cardioselective beta-blocker with a rapid onset and very short duration of action.

Give a 40 mg IV bolus over one minute. 10 ml vials containing 100 mg esmolol (10 mg/ml) do not need dilution prior to administration. Initiate maintenance infusion at 4 mg/min for four minutes. If response is inadequate, give a further 40 mg bolus and increase infusion rate to 8 mg/min. If response remains inadequate, give a further 40 mg bolus and increase infusion rate to a maximum rate of 12 mg/min.

Flecainide

Indication: For arrhythmias associated with WPW syndrome.

2 mg/kg IV or maximum 150 mg over 10–30 minutes. Maintenance infusion 1.5 mg/kg/hr (in 5% dextrose or normal saline) for one hour, subsequently reduced to 100–250 mcg/kg/hr for up to 24 hours. Maximum cumulative dose in first 24 hours: 600 mg.

Glucagon

Indication: Reversal of beta-blockade side-effects unresponsive to atropine.

50–150 mcg/kg in 5% dextrose as an IV bolus over at least one minute. If the response is not maintained, a further bolus dose may be required (or an infusion in 5% dextrose of 1–5 mg/hour).

Glyceryl trinitrate (GTN)

Indications: Treatment of angina, left ventricular failure and (occasionally) hypertensive emergencies.

50 mg in 50 ml of solution as supplied by the manufacturer. Commence infusion at 10 mcg/min (0.6 ml/hr), increasing by 10 mcg/min every 15 minutes until the desired effect is obtained. Maximum dose is 200 mcg/min (12 ml/hr). Tolerance is a problem, and interrupted regimes or an increase in dosage may be necessary if the infusion continues for more than 24 hours.

Although less easy to regulate, buccal GTN can be an alternative to IV therapy, particularly if all infusion pumps are in use.

Insulin

Indication: Hyperglycaemia.

50 units of short acting insulin (i.e. actrapid or humulin S) in 50 ml normal saline via an infusion pump to give an insulin concentration of 1 unit/ml.

BM stick	Insulin infusin rate (units/hr)
<5.0	0
5.1–8.0	1
8.1–10.0	2
10.1–13.0	3
13.1–17.0	4
17.1–20.0	6

Isoprenaline

Indications: Symptomatic bradyarrhythmias awaiting temporary pacing; reversal of beta-blockade.

5 mg in 500 ml 5% dextrose or saline to give a concentration of 10 mcg/ml, infused at 1 ml/min initially, increasing the infusion rate to maintain an adequate ventricular rate.

Isosorbide dinitrate

Indications: Treatment of angina, left ventricular failure.

50 mg in 50 ml of solution as supplied by the manufacturer. Commence infusion at 2 mg/hr (2 ml/hr), increasing by 1mg/hr every 15 minutes until the desired effect is obtained. Doses up to 20 mg/hr may occasionally be required. Tolerance is a problem, and interrupted regimes or an increase in dosage may be necessary if the infusion continues for more than 24 hours.

Labetalol

Indications: Blood pressure control in the treatment of hypertensive emergencies or acute aortic dissection.

50 mg slow IV bolus over one minute, repeated after five minutes if necessary (max. 200 mg). For continuous infusion, make up a solution of 1 mg/ml by adding 20 ml of IV labetalol (containing 200 mg) to 180 ml of 5% dextrose to make a total volume of 200 ml. Commence infusion at 15 mg/hr, and increase every 30 to 60 minutes (up to max. of 160 mg/hr) until blood pressure falls to desired level.

Lignocaine

Indication: For suppression of ventricular arrhythmias.

50 mg bolus over a few minutes, which can be repeated to a maximum of 200 mg. This is followed by an infusion of 4 mg/min for 30 minutes, 2 mg/min for two hours, then 1 mg/min for 24 hours (500 mg in 500 ml 5% dextrose, giving a concentration of 1 mg/ml).

Magnesium sulphate

Indications: For use in monomorphic and polymorphic ventricular tachycardia (especially in the presence of hypokalaemia).

10 mmol of 50% magnesium sulphate in 100 ml 5% dextrose or normal saline IV over 20 minutes, co-administered with 60 mmol of potassium chloride over two hours, if serum potassium concentration < 4.0 mmol/l.

Noradrenaline acid tartrate

Indications: A powerful alpha and beta agonist, used to increase systemic vascular resistance and so raise blood pressure in a severely hypotensive patient when other measures have failed.

4 mg (4 ml) added to 46 ml 5% dextrose for administration via syringe driver, or 40 mg in 460 ml 5% dextrose for administration via infusion pump. This gives a concentration of 80 mcg/ml. Initiate infusion at a rate of 0.16–0.33 ml/min (10–20 ml/hr), adjusting according to the pressor effect observed.

Potassium chloride

Indications: Hypokalaemia, digoxin toxicity.

Add 20 to 60 mmol to 100 ml or 250 ml 5% dextrose or normal saline, and shake infusion bag thoroughly to mix after the addition of potassium. Use a suitable infusion device so as not to infuse at a rate greater than 20 mmol/hr. Concentrated solutions may be irritant and painful, therefore administer centrally if possible, or add 2 ml of 1% lignocaine to infusate.

Sodium bicarbonate

Indication: Prolonged resuscitation.

50 ml of 8.4% solution (50 mmol) by slow intravenous injection. Do not administer via an ET tube, and avoid venous extravasation (causes tissue necrosis).

Sodium nitroprusside

Indication: Hypertensive crisis.

Add 50 mg to 500 ml 5% dextrose (concentration 100 mcg/ml). Prepare solution immediately prior to use, and protect from light during administration. Fresh solution is required every four hours, or earlier if it becomes discoloured. Normal duration of therapy should not exceed 72 hours, and should be terminated over 10–30 minutes to avoid rebound. If infused for more than 24 hours, give vitamin B_{12} (hydroxycobalamin) injection 1 mg IM. Check serum thiocyanate concentration (toxic level >100 mcg/ml) or monitor blood gases for metabolic acidosis, which occurs with cyanide toxicity and should rapidly reverse when the infusion is stopped.

Initial dose (in a patient not already taking antihypertensive treatment): 0.3 mcg/kg/min gradually increased as required to usual dosage range of 0.5–6 mcg/kg/min (max. rate is 8 mcg/kg/min). Lower doses will be required for patients already receiving antihypertensive treatment. Infusion should be discontinued after 10 minutes if there is no response.

Streptokinase

Indications: For thrombolysis in acute MI.

Ensure no contraindications are present prior to administration. For acute MI, administer 1.5 million units in 100 ml normal saline over one hour.

Verapamil

Indication: For treatment of AVNRT in patients where adenosine is contraindicated.

Verapamil is given as a slow IV injection of 5–10 mg over two minutes. After 10 minutes, a further 5 mg can be administered if required.

References

British National Formulary (34). 1997.

Opie, L. H. (1991). *Drugs for the Heart*. W.B. Saunders Company.

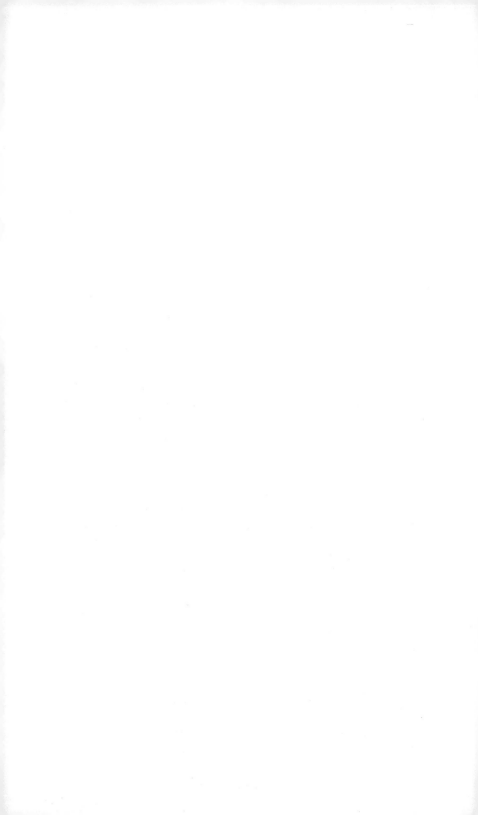

Index

ACE inhibitors, acute myocardial
infarction, 80–5
administration regime, 83–4
background, 80–2
exclusion criteria, 83
inclusion criteria, 82–3
Acute ischaemic syndromes
diagnosis, 8–17
acute myocardial infarction, 8–15
background, 8
unstable angina, 15
pathophysiology, 4–7
background, 3–4
non-Q-wave infarction, 5–6
Q-wave infarction, 6
risk factors, 4
therapeutic implications, 6
unstable angina, 5
Acute myocardial infarction
ACE inhibitors, 80–5
administration regime, 83–4
background, 80–2
exclusion criteria, 83
inclusion criteria, 82–3
arrhythmias complicating,
43–61
background, 43–5
bradyarrhythmias, 55–60
tachyarrhythmias, 45–55
beta-blocker therapy, 32–6
adverse effects, 34–5
atenolol, 34

background, 32–3
convalescent phase, 35–6
exclusion criteria, 33–4
indications for, 33
calcium antagonist therapy, 36
clinical features, 8–9
diagnosis, 8–15
electrocardiographic signs, 9–15
emergency and early care, 18–23
background, 18
cardiac care unit, 20–2
emergency care, 19–20
hyperglycaemia, 21–2
hypokalaemia, 20–1
magnesium therapy, 21
nitrate therapy, 21
pre-existing drug therapy, 22
prophylactic antiarrhythmic
therapy, 22
and hypertension, 135–6
in-hospital convalescence, 91–4
background, 91
late ventricular arrhythmias, 93
left ventricular aneurysm, 93
post-infarction pericarditis, 92
recurrent ischaemia, 92–3
thromboembolic complications,
91–2
mechanical complications,
86–90
background, 86
mitral regurgitation, 87–9

ventricular fibrillation, 53
ventricular tachyarrhythmias,
  49–50
Asystole, 63–5
Atenolol, 34, 134
Atrial fibrillation, 47–9, 112–15
Atrial flutter, 115–17
Atrial tachycardia, 124
Atrioventricular node re-entry
  tachycardia, 117–20
Atropine, 173–4

Beta-blockers, acute myocardial
  infarction, 32–6
adverse effects, 34–5
atenolol, 34
background, 32–3
convalescent phase, 35–6
exclusion criteria, 33–4
indications for, 33
Bradyarrhythmias, 55–60, 130
first degree heart block, 55
Mobitz type I second degree block,
  55–7
Mobitz type II second degree block,
  58, 59
sinus bradycardia and sinus arrest,
  55
third degree (complete) block,
  58–60
Bradycardia, 55
Bretylium tosylate, 174
Bundle of Kent, 120

Calcium antagonists, acute
  myocardial infarction, 36
Calcium chloride/gluconate, 174
Cardiac tamponade, 153
Cardiogenic shock, 74–9
background, 74–5
diagnosis, 75–6
hypotension, 77–8
left ventricular dysfunction, 76
mechanical complications, 77
right ventricular dysfunction, 76–7

Central venous cannulation, 160–3
internal jugular cannulation, 161–2
subclavian cannulation, 160–1
Chest pain, 15–17
Convalescence, 91–4
background, 91
left ventricular aneurysm, 93
left ventricular arrhythmias, 93
post-infarction pericarditis, 92
recurrent ischaemia, 92–3
thromboembolic complications,
  91–2
Coronary artery bypass grafting, 41
Coronary care unit, 1–3
acute myocardial infarction, 20–2
hyperglycaemia, 21–2
hypokalaemia, 20–1
magnesium therapy, 21
nitrate therapy, 21
pre-existing drug therapy, 22
prophylactic antiarrhythmic
  therapy, 22
background, 1–2
guidelines for admission, 2–3

DC cardioversion, 169–70
Diagnosis of acute ischaemic
  syndromes, 8–17
acute myocardial infarction, 8–16
background, 8
unstable angina, 15
Digibind, 174
Digoxin, 174–5
toxicity, 156–7
Dobutamine, 175
Dopamine, 176

Eclampsia, 136–7
Ectopic beats, 45–6
Electrocardiography, 9–15 see also
  individual conditions
Electromechanical dissociation, 65–6
Esmolol, 176–7

Flecainide, 177

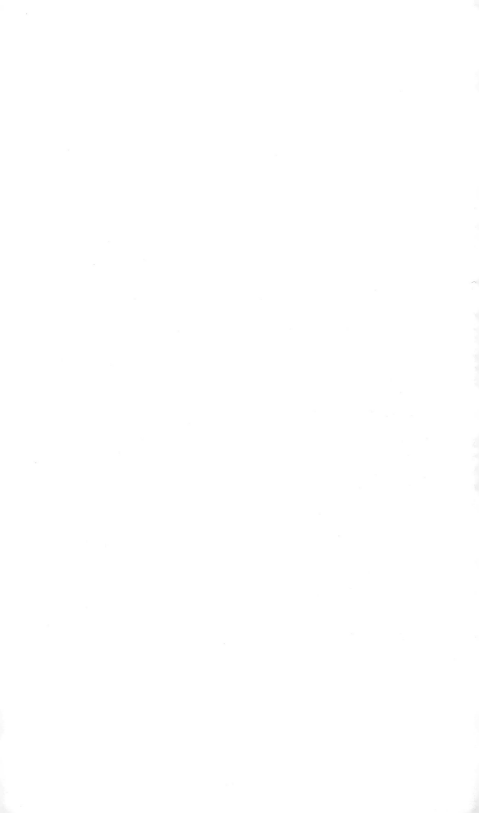